SURVIVING
TEEN PREGNANCY

SURVIVING
TEEN PREGNANCY
Your Choices, Dreams,
and Decisions

By Shirley Arthur

Illustrated by Perry Bergman

Revised Edition

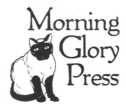

Morning
Glory
Press

Buena Park, California

Library of Congress Cataloging-in-Publication Data
Arthur, Shirley, 1951-
    Surviving teen pregnancy : your choices, dreams, and decisions /
by Shirley Arthur; illustrated by Perry Bergman. — Rev. ed.
        p.   cm.
    Includes bibliographical references and index.
    Summary: A guide for pregnant adolescents in making decisions,
getting help, planning the future, and, generally, surviving.
    ISBN 1-885356-05-6. — ISBN 1-885356-06-4 (pbk.)
    1. Teenage mothers—United States—Juvenile literature.
  2. Teenage pregnancy—United States—Juvenile literature.
  3. Teenage mothers—United States—Life skills guides—Juvenile
literature. 4. Unmarried mothers—United States—Juvenile literature.   [1. Pregnancy. 2. Teenage mothers. 3. Unmarried
mothers.]   I. Title
    HQ759.4.A78   1996
    306.85'6—dc20   95-33735
                                                              CIP
                                                              AC

MORNING GLORY PRESS, INC.
6595 San Haroldo Way   Buena Park, CA 90620
(714) 828-1998 FAX (714) 828-2049
Printed and bound in the United States of America

Contents

Preface   9

Foreword   11

Part One

JUST A LITTLE BIT PREGNANT   14

1   Are You Really Pregnant?   36

Do you think you're pregnant?; Discussing your
options; What is not an option?; Getting medical help;
Getting emotional help; Other problems; Abuse; Are
you a runaway?; Drug use; What will happen to you?

2   You Are Not Alone   48

Carol's story; Michelle, the last girl anyone thought
would get pregnant; Kim, too; The same problem; What
are you feeling?; How pregnancy affects your emotions;
Good nutrition; What can you do?

3   Taking Care of You and Your Baby   60

Special needs of teen mothers; Nutrition; How much
should you gain?; What about junk food?; Exercise
helps; Smoking, drinking, drugs; Preparing for childbirth; Your appearance; Taking care of yourself.

Part Two
MAKING CHOICES   68

4   Abortion—A Difficult Choice   71
What is abortion?; How is it done?; What does it cost?;
Is it painful?; Will you be depressed—or worse?; Where
should you go if you want an abortion?; Will they tell
anyone?; Risks and side effects; Pros and cons; Questions to ask yourself; Is it too late for this option?

5   Adoption Is an Option   80
Closed adoption; Open adoption; Choosing an
agency; Independent adoption; Rights of baby's father;
What if I change my mind?; What will it cost?; Pros
and cons; Questions to ask yourself; Adoption isn't easy.

6   Choosing Active Parenting   92
What are your options?; Keeping baby and staying
single; Parenting; What about baby's father?; Getting
married; Weighing the good and the bad; Why is the
"con" list longer?; Questions to ask yourself.

7   It's *Your* Decision   104
How do you decide?; Don't give decision power away;
It's *your* decision; Others are affected; Your baby; Your
parents and family; Your friends; Your boyfriend; Listen
to your fantasies; Role-play your choices; What would
you do if . . . ?; Put yourself in the future; If it hurts, is it
wrong?; What if you decide wrong?

Part Two
WRITING YOUR LIFE SCRIPT   116

8   Social Insecurity—Boyfriends and Others   119
Jennifer; What should Jennifer do?; Your friends; Your
boyfriend; What if you decide to say goodbye?;
Inquiring minds want to know; When smart people ask
stupid questions; Talking can help.

9   Money Matters   130
Handling baby costs; If you're living with parents; If
you're getting married; Child care; Learning to budget;
Public aid; Child support?; Can you afford school?; One
day at a time.

10   Birth Control Means Life Control   140
Are you a sexual person?; Handling your sexuality;
Should you be in love?; Birth control; These won't
prevent pregnancy; Sex isn't always planned; Making
birth control work.

11   Getting What You Want   154
A job can build self-esteem; What can you be?; Education is important; Four steps to what you want; Sometimes you need a little help; A little healthy competition;
Get started on your future.

12   Following Your Dreams   166
The joy of making choices; Tools to help you; Meditation; Movies for the mind; See your past differently;
Picturing your future; Self-talk; You've been given a
challenge; How do you know when you're "there"?

Appendix   179
Annotated Bibliography   181
Index   189

Acknowledgments

I'd like to thank Jeanne Lindsay, President and Editor of Morning Glory Press, for taking a chance on this book, and for her advice and assistance. I'd also like to thank the young women who share their thoughts in this book, especially the young women at Bridgeway House and George Washington High School in Denver.

My husband, Jay, showed me that it's possible to write a book and get it published, and gave encouragement, advice, and patience while I researched and wrote.

I owe my parents a great debt for standing by me years ago and supporting me (literally and figuratively) while I got my life together.

Thank you, Kristina and Kelly, for your inspiration and patience, even when you didn't know that you were providing it.

Preface

We've all heard that more than a million teenagers get pregnant every year. It's been called a national tragedy. When a teenager finds out that she's pregnant, she doesn't feel like there are a million young women just like her. It doesn't feel like a national tragedy, it feels like a personal one. Her world changes suddenly, and those changes touch the lives of everyone she knows and loves.

Pregnancy isn't an end, but a beginning. Sometimes it's the beginning of maturity, of adult decision-making, of responsibility. There is such a thing as self-fulfilling prophecy. If pregnant teens are told that they'll live in poverty, they probably will. If they're told that they don't have much of a future, then they probably won't. Since they can't go back and change the past, wouldn't it be nice if they could control their future? They could get on with their lives, make plans and goals like everyone else, and enjoy life.

We all define our lives around challenges that are given to us. Teen pregnancy is a challenge.

I waited to write this book until I was sure that my daughter and I had both survived my teen pregnancy. I realized later that we had survived all along. Survival doesn't always mean happiness. It doesn't mean there won't be challenges. It doesn't mean that other people will always be happy for you.

Survival doesn't mean we make *all* the right choices, but that we make our choices right. Being a survivor makes you feel good about yourself.

Shirley Arthur
January, 1996

Foreword

In the past several years, the devastating consequences of premature pregnancy and adolescent parenting have been well documented in the research and in the media. Yet, we who work in the field continue to encounter the success stories—those who have made it—where the personalization of poverty, hopelessness, and children with special needs is not the scenario of a number of teen parents.

They are working, productive, and happy, and their children are well adjusted and achieving. Somehow they had a vision of how a caring family could be, looked at their choices, and made decisions which lifted them above the norm. At a very personal level they possess the dedication, knowledge, and skills which prevent them from becoming part of the cold, hard, and impersonal statistics we so often hear.

From my experience in working with pregnant and parenting teens the past nineteen years, I have found many of them full of hope and anticipation for what lies ahead. They dream of independence, a successful marriage, a good paying job, a nice home, and children of whom they can be proud. They optimistically expect that all of these things will happen for them.

Unfortunately, however, only a few have developed a plan of action or have the skills and knowledge needed to make these dreams become a reality. They need assistance in identifying and working through the specific decisions which will empower them to take control of their lives.

In *Surviving Teen Pregnancy*, Shirley Arthur has given pregnant and parenting teens a plan and a process. The book is written from her personal experiences as a teen parent, and in a language and format which will appeal to these young women.

Shirley knows what decisions must be made, and how teenagers are likely to approach each decision. She is sensitive to the practical as well as the emotional roadblocks which may keep a young woman from achieving her goals. Shirley discusses these as a friend, someone who cares about her reader's future. She does not preach, but explores the alternatives with them, respectful of their ability to make their own decisions.

I think a majority of the young women with whom I work will find this book a breath of fresh air. It does not dwell on the problems teens face, but instead offers a blueprint for turning these challenges into tools for achieving maturity and developing a positive and satisfying life. I foresee young women not only reading this book early in their pregnancy, but referring to it time and time again as they begin to identify and struggle with each critical issue.

Surviving Teen Pregnancy is upbeat, and it lets teens know they can succeed. It should be available for all teens who even suspect they might be pregnant, for their partners, their friends, and others who care about young people.

Sue Dolezal
Teen Renaissance Program Director
Brighton School District 27J
Brighton, Colorado

To Kristina and Kelly

. . . Thank you for being my daughters.

And, to Jay for his encouragement.

Introduction PART ONE

JUST A LITTLE BIT PREGNANT

I lay on the grass on my stomach that warm, sunny autumn day over 20 years ago. I felt something flutter across my lower abdomen, the fleeting ripple of something trying to grab my attention. I was fascinated for a brief moment, waiting for the flutter again. Another quick flutter. Suddenly, I was gripped with a fright that sent my mind spinning and made the ground where I was lying and the trees and sky—everything—seem unreal.

I sat up to try to calm myself. Although shivering with cold, I was drenched in sweat, my heart was beating wildly in my chest, and I was shaking. "It's true," I thought. "I'm pregnant." What I meant was, "I'm doomed."

Nearly six months earlier I had broken up with Tom (not his real name). I was sixteen and he was a year older. All I could think of was to get back together with him somehow,

and at least I wouldn't be in this alone. Then he'd have to
take part of the blame. I worried that he'd think it wasn't
his, or that he'd say he hadn't seen me for a long time.

It wasn't that I was shocked to find myself pregnant. I
couldn't believe it, that's all. I had thought that something
would protect me, like my young age, or my religion, or my
plan that I wouldn't have a family until I was at least
twenty-five.

There had been plenty of clues: the throwing up every
morning for two months, the mysterious dizzy spells, my
swelling waist that I attributed to peanut butter and jelly
sandwiches, my growing breasts which I credited to my
desire for large breasts.

In school, we had sex education classes every year. They
separated the classes by gender, showed films, and then had
a question-and-answer period. I knew that sexual activity
causes pregnancy. What confused me was being told by
one instructor that it would not be difficult to put a stop to
his advances. "He has much stronger sexual urges than you
do. Women do not respond the way men do, and that is
why it is up to you to say no."

I waited for the "real woman" in me to become disgusted
with the whole process and put a stop to it. I talked to a
girlfriend who had been dating her boyfriend for nearly two
years. Although I was too shy to talk about my situation
with her, I probed her to talk about her relationship.

"Sometimes," she told me, "we go park and I take off
my shirt and let him touch them. We do that for hours
sometimes and end up getting in a fight because he wants
me to undress the rest of the way and I won't."

I pretended to be shocked. "You do that?" I asked.
"What keeps you from undressing all the way?"

"Are you kidding?" she said. "It's disgusting. Sometimes
I can't stand it when he tries to kiss my boobs—I just want

to keep him happy enough so he doesn't go out with some-one else. I'm not having sex 'til I'm married and have to."

That clinched it for me. Something was really wrong with me. Not only was I not fighting him to leave my clothes on, but I found myself disappointed if he wanted to go home instead of parking.

I knew it was my responsibility to stop it, and I had every intention of doing so. I would stand in front of the mirror in my bedroom, clench my fists, and chant over and over again: "I will not let him touch me, I will not let him touch me." Then of course when we went out and I put up no resistance, I would go home, cry, and feel guilty and worthless.

I decided not to worry so much. After all, he didn't seem worried. I wasn't like the girl in study hall who wrote dirty words on her notebook and dyed her hair about five differ-ent colors. Everyone said she would get pregnant. Nobody said that about me. They wrote "You're so sweet" in my yearbook. "Sweet" people didn't get pregnant. If I could hang on for a couple of years, we could marry and all my problems would be over.

It started getting tougher to hang on to our relationship. He became self-involved and uncaring. He stopped taking me out. He became distant and cold and made terrible comments about me in front of his friends. I cried almost every time we went out. I carried around a heavy, hurt feeling in my chest.

*He was suddenly a little boy
afraid of getting caught,
and he was ready to run.*

When I missed my period, I became a master at making excuses. I decided to give myself three extra weeks because it was summer and hot and my body probably was adjusting. Then, I gave myself three extra weeks for "nerves." I told Tom about it and we decided to wait and see. The frightened look on his face disturbed me. He was suddenly a little boy afraid of getting caught and he was ready to run. Suddenly, I wanted to protect him.

That summer, he went out of state to visit friends. He was to be gone for a month and promised to write. I went to the mail box every day looking for a letter, but it never came.

When he returned, I still had not had my period, but I decided to tell him that everything was okay. Obviously, he was acting so odd because he was frightened. He was relieved and joyful when I told him I wasn't pregnant.

"Yes," I said, "I was so happy, too." Then I would think, well, I *will* be happy when I start my period. The thought of being pregnant was unthinkable to me. Even the thought of being married was unthinkable.

So, although I was throwing up nearly every morning, was tired most of the time, had dizzy spells, and most important, had no periods, I refused to believe or even think that I might be pregnant. I read what books I could find to reassure myself that I was merely suffering from a case of the nerves. "The mind does strange things," I read in more than one book. "It can trick your periods into stopping." Obviously, my mind was doing strange things.

Soon I heard that Tom was seeing someone else on the sly. Actually, he was seeing her openly. I just *thought* he was being sly. I found out who she was and all I could about her. I walked past her house and tried to seek her out at school to see what she looked like. He quit calling.

I had to admit that we would no longer see each other—and yet, I never really admitted it. I became depressed and walked through each day in a cloud of misery. My surroundings seemed unreal, and I stopped caring about school. I had ignored my friends for so long that I had no one to talk to.

---

*The thought of having some terrible disease
frightened me, but not as much
as the thought of being pregnant.*

Although I kept reassuring myself that I was *not* pregnant, I had a nagging fear in the back of my mind. I convinced myself that I had some incurable disease, like cancer. It explained why I felt so tired all the time and why I didn't have periods anymore.

The thought of having some terrible disease frightened me, but not as much as the thought of being pregnant. I imagined that people would stick by me if I was sick. I even fantasized my funeral.

As I lay on the grass that day in the park and felt the baby stirring inside me, I knew. It was a moment of clarity and insight, as if God had decided that I was ready to know, and He opened a giant door and let me peer inside at my future. I was frightened beyond belief. My mind spun trying to decide what to do. I was not going to die. I was going to have a baby.

I decided that I would go away. I didn't know where I would go or what I would do, but I knew that I could not stay at home. I imagined myself living somewhere with my baby, taking care of both of us.

I floated through the next few days on a cloud of fear and hopelessness. I could think of no one in whom I could confide, no saviour. I tried to call Tom. I called his house many times only to have his parents tell me with more and more anger that he was *not* home, and finally, that even if he was home, he had no desire to talk to me. I gave up.

Finally, I confided in a girlfriend who I had not talked to in a few months. She came to my house and I spilled it all out in a rush of tears.

"Oh, don't worry," she said. "It happened to my big sister and no one ever knew."

"What did she do?" I asked.

"I don't know exactly, something to make her period come—but I'll ask her."

I anxiously waited while she phoned her sister. When my friend came back, she was annoyed that her sister thought that it was *she* who needed the information. Apparently she had to convince her sister that it was a friend and not her.

"Well?" I asked anxiously.

"She said to try drinking a whole quart of gin. We don't even have to go buy it; she has some left."

That night was spent in my friend's bathroom, drinking out of a bottle of cheap gin, taking alternate hot and cold baths, throwing up, and waiting for the promised period. It never came.

The next day my friend and I nursed hangovers and dwelled on my situation.

"I don't know what to tell you," she said. "I guess you're in a mess now."

---

*The thought of telling my parents
was enough to make me
wake up at night in terror.*

I thought about suicide. I daydreamed about it. At that moment, death seemed to be the only way out. Everyone would cry and miss me, and no one would ever know about the baby. I could imagine Tom missing me and being sorry that he had hurt me. The only drawback was that I would be dead—and I did *not* want to be dead. It was to be the last time I considered suicide.

I was not afraid of having the baby or even of caring for the baby. However, the thought of telling my parents was enough to make me wake up at night in terror. When would I tell them? During a commercial while watching Twilight Zone on TV? On the way out of the house in the morning? "I'm going to school now, and oh, by the way, I'm pregnant." I knew I couldn't do it. I tried several times, and couldn't get the words out.

I would have the baby, and we would survive—somehow.

I knew that the situation was becoming critical. I already looked pregnant, could not fit into my clothes, and felt teachers' and students' eyes glaring at my swollen stomach. I managed to hide my condition from my parents by wearing baggy clothes and avoiding them.

I packed my bags. I had read about a home in a large town about 400 miles away. I would go there and wait until the baby was born. I would no longer have a family. I would start a new life. I had just enough money for the bus fare—$12.00.

For some reason, mysterious even to me, I decided that I had to finish out the following week in school. I had mid-term exams that week, and I felt that I needed to stay for them.

I decided to talk to my friend and tell her that I was leaving town. "Look," she said, "I guess my idea didn't work. I feel real bad about that. I found out that my sister really had an abortion! She saved up the $1200 and went to New York. It's not legal, but it's a good doctor—safer than going to Mexico."

"It might as well be a million," I said to her. I had not thought of abortion. Suddenly, a ray of hope! An abortion! No one would know. I would go away quietly, and when I came back, it would be as if I had never been pregnant. But, where would I get $1200?

"Don't even think about it," my friend said. "You're too far along. I asked my sister. I'm sorry."

"It's not your fault," I said.

"You have to tell someone," she said. "I work afternoons for a social worker. Would you go talk to her?"

"I don't know," I said. "I already decided to go away."

"Well, just talk to her first."

She insisted, so I went with her that afternoon and found myself waiting in a small, dreary office. There was a mother there with her five small, dirty children. The office smelled of poverty and hopelessness.

"I don't belong here," I kept telling myself. "This is a welfare office."

I waited an hour and a half. Finally, I was called into a smaller, drearier office. Across the desk sat a woman who looked like someone's grandmother.

"So," she began. "You're pregnant?" I was amazed how easy it was for her to say.

I was relieved that my friend had already told her. I just didn't think I could get the words out. It was frightening thinking about being pregnant, but it was terrifying speaking out loud about it. My face reddened and burned. I started crying, and getting anything out of me was hopeless. The grandmotherly lady rolled her chair around to my side of the desk and proceeded to rub my back.

"It'll be okay," she said. "A year from now, you'll look back and it'll be all over."

Finally, she told me that she would have to inform my parents. I felt trapped. Would my parents disown me?

Would I be homeless and poor the rest of my life? I had already gotten an inkling of people's stares and whispers.

Some small window of wisdom in my mind told me that I could not leave town; there was no running away. I would have to stay and face the music. I knew that the nice grandmotherly lady from Social Services would pay a visit to my house and bring the distressing news to my family.

I found my mother crying in the living room.
I hadn't counted on that.
I had expected raging anger, but not grief.

The next day I was too upset to go to school, so I left the house and wandered all day. I went to the park, to the library, and to McDonald's for lunch. It was the longest day of my life. When I went home at 4:00, I found my mother crying in the living room. I hadn't counted on that. I had expected raging anger, but not grief. It was harder for me to deal with than anger.

My sister was cooking dinner in the kitchen, fried chicken and mashed potatoes and the whole bit. I wondered who was going to feel like eating all that food. I had an urge to walk in and punch her for being so good and never causing any trouble. I knew that wouldn't go over, so I shot her a dirty look, as if she somehow had gotten me into this mess.

We waited for my father to come home so we could tell him. It was a long wait. Being one of the first advocates of the "Just Say No" technique of birth control, all he could say was, "Don't you know how to say no?"

I wanted to tell him, "*I don't remember any question that I could say no to,*" but I knew he'd think I was being smartmouthed. Then, I thought of telling them that I'd been raped, but I remembered that I told the social worker that Tom was the father.

*It was a nightmarish prospect
for the parents of a son that he could be saddled
with monthly child support payments
for eighteen years.*

The social worker also told Tom's parents, and all hell
broke loose. To my surprise, he did not deny it. His parents' concern was that I would try to collect child support. I
hadn't thought anything about money. I don't think I'd ever
heard the word "support" used when talking about money.
It was a nightmarish prospect for the parents of a son that
he could be saddled with monthly child support payments
for eighteen years.

Having a baby was expensive, I was told, and insurance
did not cover pregnancy unless the mother was married. I
kept thinking how odd it was that you had to *pay* to go
through all this. I was bringing financial hardship to my
family. Not only to my family, but potentially to *his* family.
I wanted to be left alone to handle my situation, but I could
not. I had no money, no support system outside my family.

Relieved that at last I wasn't keeping secrets, I decided
to go hide in my room and stay there for the duration of the
pregnancy. I became fearful of leaving the house, of having
people see me, even of having someone come to the house.
Every ring of the telephone, every strange voice in the
house sent adrenaline rushing and left me shaking and
drained.

My parents had no idea how to guide me. They never
talked about me leaving the house. I believe that they
secretly wished (as I did) that Tom would come up to the
door one day, bearing flowers, and ask me to marry him.

Although I'd always thought that marriage wouldn't be
that great, it seemed the ideal, easy way out. He would

grow to love me and our child the way I believed I loved him. It was more a way to get out of the house, away from the humiliation of being pregnant and having to live with my parents. Like most other teenagers, I looked forward to the day I would be independent and living on my own.

One day he came to the door. My heart leapt with fear when I heard the doorbell. My mom came to get me, telling me who it was. A feeling of relief swept over me, and I felt that everything would be okay. He would take care of both of us. I would have no ugly decisions to make.

I tried to make myself as presentable as possible. I was wearing my mother's maternity clothes which were out of date.

My parents left us alone on the sofa. Neither of us talked for about ten minutes. Finally, he told me he was sorry about all this and I could call him any time to talk.

"Why are you here?" I asked.

"Actually," he said, "my mom thought I should come and talk to you about something."

"What?"

"We all think it's best if you give the baby to a good home—you know, where it has two good parents. People who adopt always have lots of money it'd be better off."

"Wouldn't that make you feel a little bit bad?" I asked.

He thought for a minute. "I guess if it turns out to be a boy. I always thought I'd like to have a son."

I noticed how young he looked,
like a little boy.

I was heartbroken. I went back to my room and cried. My mother anxiously asked how the talk went.

"He just wanted me to give the baby up for adoption," I told her. I wasn't sure what I wanted.

After a few days, the social worker came back to visit me. I sat quietly on the sofa next to her. She talked about adoptive parents, how good the homes were, and how well they were screened. I was extremely depressed and could not even talk to her.

She began talking louder and louder as if I could not hear her, and I knew that she was getting irritated with my lack of response. I sensed that she wanted to grab me by the shoulders and shake some response out of me. I just shrugged at her.

I retreated back to my bedroom to eat peanut butter and jelly sandwiches and read. While everyone in the family was nervous and anxious for me to make some kind of decision, I decided that I had plenty of time, that I would let things flow along as they had been. I was afraid of hurting my parents again. My mother changed between wanting me to keep the baby and, because of my age, saying that perhaps I should give the baby to an adoptive family. As she changed, my decision changed.

Each time that I thought I had made an intelligent, final decision, everything tossed around in my head and soon made no sense at all. There seemed no "right" way out of the mess I had created. The days slowed down so that each day seemed a week long. I wasn't really upset anymore. It seemed like small things, like a good TV show or reading the paper, made me happy. I could have lived that way forever.

I was being carried down some long river against my control.

I had a teacher for the home-bound. Pregnant girls could not go to public school at that time, and this teacher was becoming increasingly frustrated with me. I was distant and depressed. She helped me as best she could and walked me through tests to help me keep my grades up.

My older sister helped, coaxing me to an occasional movie. But, as I realized later, my pregnancy was difficult for her, too; I could hide at home from the questions and stares from the other kids at school, but she could not.

By the beginning of my eighth month of pregnancy, I still had not made a decision concerning the baby. I had been to the doctor, but did not have any plans on what hospital to go to, nor had I given it much thought. I was being carried down some long river against my control. I knew there was a waterfall at the end, but I wasn't sure what I'd find at the bottom.

We were alone, it seemed,
and the baby seemed to be the last thing
that I had to look forward to.

In the doctor's office, a local obstetrician, I occasionally saw another girl obviously in the same condition as I. She looks so young, I would think, too young to have a baby. Somehow I pictured myself being more mature than this young, scared girl sitting across from me in that office.

I found myself becoming more attached to the creature swimming inside me. We were alone, it seemed, and the baby seemed to be the last thing that I had to look forward to. I imagined the baby doll-like and lovable and someone to finally love me back. Permanently.

Then one day, a friend of my mother came to visit. She had had a baby a year before and was bringing her baby clothes over for me. My mother left them in my room, in a box, where they stayed untouched for a couple of weeks. Then one day, I took them all out and looked at them, touched each tiny T-shirt and fleece nightgown. I knew then that I would keep the baby. I thought a little about money, how the baby would feel about growing up without a father, about how my parents would feel, and about how hard it would be. But I based my decision on something more basic, like the fleecy touch of a tiny nightgown.

When my mother saw the baby clothes put away in the dresser and questioned me, she learned what my decision was. My parents took responsibility for such details as where the baby was to be born, and where the money would come from.

I was much older before I realized the magnitude of these tasks, and the obvious stress on my whole family. And his. His family would pay for medical expenses in return for release of future responsibility.

He called me just once, to let me know his distress that his parents made him sell his van to cover the medical expenses.

"I'm so sorry," I said in a fit of ignorance. "I wish I could help, but I don't have any money."

They forgot to tell me that childbirth is painful. My daughter was born on February 13th, a few minutes before midnight. "Can't you put down her birthday as the 14th?" I asked. But there was to be no breaking the rules, no stretching the truth. We would have to tell things as they were. "I guess I should have waited," I said.

"Possibly ten years," the doctor said.

I really didn't see my baby until the next morning. That morning, beginning about 9:00, the nurses began bringing the babies to their respective mothers. When they didn't bring mine, I questioned the nurse. She looked startled.

"You don't really want to hold the baby, do you?" she questioned.

"Yeah," I said. "The other mothers got their babies."

"Just a minute," she said, and she rushed from the room.

After about ten minutes, she returned holding my baby.

"I'm sorry," she said. "You are so young I didn't think you were keeping the baby." She handed me the baby, kind of clucked her tongue, and said, "Good luck."

A friend of mine had told me that newborns are ugly. I braced myself for my first glimpse of the baby. My friend was wrong. When I first looked at the tiny bundle lying in my arms, she looked up at me with bright blue eyes and the sweetest little face I had ever seen. I was instantly in love. I unwrapped her blankets and touched the soft baby skin and counted all her fingers and toes. I felt a rush of love and feeling for her. I was elated.

My mother was my only visitor,
and there were no flowers,
cards of congratulations,
or excited phone calls from friends.

The next day, however, I was less than elated. I was in a ward, which meant there were three other mothers in the room with me. I had suffered through two "visiting hours" which meant that I went out into the lobby to read magazines while the other mothers visited with husbands and friends. My mother was my only visitor, and there were no flowers, cards of congratulations, or excited phone calls from friends.

During my pregnancy I had a fantasy that Tom would come to the hospital after the birth. After seeing her in the nursery, he would fall head over heels in love with me. He would then carry us both off into the sunset and take care of us.

Unfortunately, my hospital bed was by the door of the ward and near the elevators. Every time I heard the elevator doors opening and closing and footsteps walking toward the ward, my heart went into my throat. But it was always someone else's husband, brother, or friend.

By the second day in the hospital, I had sunk into a deep depression. On the third morning, I was desperate to leave. That morning I was agitated and depressed. The woman who sold papers every day ambled through the ward with her newspapers, magazines, and candy. I did not realize that you had to *pay* for these things. I thought, "How nice that the hospital would do this for the patients."

"I'll have a paper," I said as she pushed her cart by me.

She handed me the paper and stood there while I opened it and began reading.

"That'll be fifteen cents," she said.

I looked at her and immediately (but quietly) began to cry.

She looked shocked. "What's the matter?" she asked anxiously.

"I don't have fifteen cents," I sobbed.

She shook her head, took back the paper, and continued her tour of the room. By now, every mother in the room was looking at me. I had imagined (probably correctly) that I was the talk of the floor, that the other mothers talked about me when I left the room, and that the other nurses discussed my "case" when they took their coffee breaks.

When my mother came to visit later that day, my eyes were red and swollen from crying.

"I didn't have fifteen cents for the paper," I said.

She just looked at me, wondering why I was worrying about not having fifteen cents when I had much more enormous problems. But all I could think about that day was that I did not have a penny to my name, I was totally dependent on my parents, and I might never be able to go to college and live a normal life like other people. I'd be living with my parents forever.

Finally we were home, and I started the job of caring for a newborn and getting my strength back so that I could return to high school. A couple of friends who had stood by me came to visit, and they seemed excited about the baby. Relatives either stayed away or self-consciously dropped by, not knowing whether to congratulate me or offer condolences. Most of them talked to my mother and ignored me.

"How is she doing?" they would ask.

I'm tired, I would think. I don't remember what my mother answered because I usually went to my room, which I shared with my baby. This was the only place I could be alone (with the baby, of course).

I was excited and proud as most parents are, and when I looked at her, I felt a rush of love and admiration at how pretty she was. But, I was tired.

I hadn't thought much about who would watch the baby while I went back to work or school.

My mother and I agreed that I would have responsibility for her care, and that's how I wanted it. But sometimes in the middle of the night she would wake up and cry. I would feed her, but she would stay awake crying for something I didn't seem able to give her.

I felt I couldn't catch up with my emotions. I would have paid a million dollars for a day off. I found out that caring for an infant is a constant job, and you don't have much time to reflect on *your* needs, on recovering from childbirth, on recovering emotionally, much less trying to deal with other people.

There were some things I had failed to think about during my pregnancy. For instance, I hadn't thought much about who would watch the baby while I went back to work or school. Fortunately, my mother was able to babysit for me for a few hours a day. I also had younger sisters who would occasionally babysit for me. Sometimes though, nobody was available, and I had to pay for a babysitter or stay home.

I discovered I had lost the part of my freedom that used to let me take a nap whenever I wanted to, or go for a walk, or run quickly to the store. I had another person to think about. I had a baby.

I was a mother, but I still wanted
all the things that being a teenager
was supposed to offer.

I stayed in my room and thought about my situation. I faced returning to school after six weeks, and I was terrified. I was an unwed mother (thank God we no longer use that term). Surely, I was not like the girls in the movie I had seen about a home for unwed mothers. They were all wild, promiscuous, or stupid and childlike, or they were victims of incest.

The thought terrified me, yet the thought of not returning to school terrified me even more. I did *not* want to be a dropout; in fact, I wanted to go to college. I had always gotten good grades and liked school. I had dreams of doing something exciting with my life. But, I had become afraid of leaving the house, of going out in public where people stared at me and (I knew) talked about me and my situation. I did not want to be remembered as "that girl who had the baby."

I was a mother, but I still wanted all the things that being a teenager was supposed to offer. I wanted happy school times and pretty clothes. I wanted what every girl wants. I wanted to be popular. I wanted to be prom queen.

I fantasized that when I went back, the kids would welcome me with open arms.

I was afraid of going to school, of facing the kids and the teachers. But I went back. After a few days answering questions from curious students, teachers and counselors, my days evolved into an endless routine of school, child-care, studying, and working.

I made mistakes, little slips back into childhood, like the time I forgot to pick my daughter up from the babysitter. I just forgot that I had a child. I'd throw little fits sometimes at home about not wanting to live there anymore.

One night, two years later, after getting my first college grade report, I finally realized that I was going to make it. I walked home from school on that cool, clear night, looked up at the stars, and saw my past and my future with sudden clarity.

"He's not coming back," I said softly to myself. "He's not coming back and it doesn't matter." I felt strangely peaceful and calm for the first time in two years. Why? I had *wanted* him to come back. Suddenly it seemed right that he wasn't going to help me. Knowing he wasn't coming back meant that there would be no more waiting—for *anybody*. I had myself, my family, and my daughter. I could choose to be any kind of person I wanted to be.

The thought came slowly, but I repeated it over and over. It was simple, yet seemed so important, like an earth-shattering revelation to me. "Just because I don't have a boyfriend doesn't mean I'm alone. Just because I have a baby doesn't mean I don't have a future."

Eighteen years later, I stood in my daughter's college dorm room. I was about to leave her there to begin her college life, and I was the one with a bad case of separation anxiety. I was stalling around, not really wanting to leave her in that small crowded room.

It's not the way I thought I'd feel. I thought I'd be cheering and saying hello to my freedom again. Party time! Over the years, people told me that when she was grown, I'd still be young, and I'd get a chance to live my teenage years. They didn't tell me that I wouldn't want to. Maybe I never missed anything.

How did she turn into the beautiful, self-confident, college student with what seemed like a million friends? The odds were against it. Sometimes, people would tell me that I gave up a lot to be her mother. The fact is, she gave up a lot to be my daughter.

She gave back more to me than I gave to her. I want to ask her forgiveness for the fact that she had to work for her clothes during high school, for the time my friends wanted to give her a sip of beer and I laughed along instead of protecting her, for the times I resented staying home with her instead of going to a party, for the time I told a new friend that she was my little sister, for the time I bought new shoes for myself instead of for her . . .

"Do you need anything?" I asked her.

"Yeah," she said. "Would you run to the grocery store for chips and pop?"

"Sure."

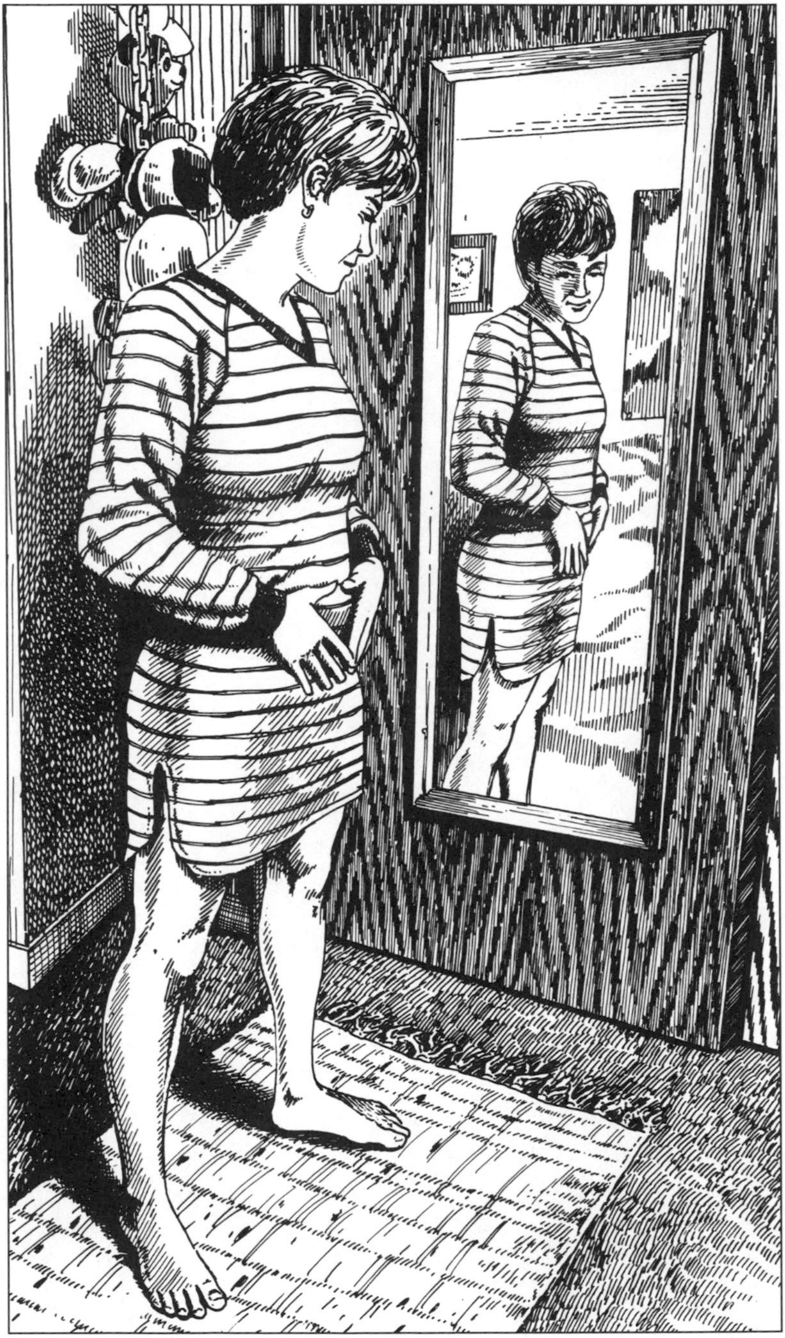

CHAPTER 1

ARE YOU REALLY PREGNANT?

Pregnant (preg-nent) adj. Fr. 1: Containing unborn young within the body. 2: Abounding in fancy, wit, or resourcefulness. 3: Having possibilities of development or consequence.   —Webster

It's scary to say the word aloud when you think you might be pregnant. You either think you're pregnant, or know you are. Maybe you're making excuses to make yourself feel better:

Maybe it's just the flu.

Maybe I'm infertile, and that's why I haven't had a period.

I've never been regular anyway.

It's just nerves.

I must have miscounted.

*I've never had regular periods. I read somewhere
that if you exercise a lot, sometimes your periods stop.
That's what I thought it was.*

Donna, pregnant at 17

If you think you might be pregnant, it's better to know
for sure. If you've already revealed your pregnancy, you
need guidance on what to do now. Chances are your family
is just as upset and confused as you are. That's not much
help when you need guidance.

If you haven't found out for sure that you're pregnant, if
you suspect you are and don't know what to do, please get
a pregnancy test immediately. Don't wait for a missed
period or for early pregnancy symptoms to go away. A
missed period doesn't always mean you're pregnant. Some
young women have light periods when they're pregnant.

*When I realized I was pregnant, I was scared. I
didn't want to tell my boyfriend. I was more scared to
tell him than I was my mother. I thought if I told him,
he'd probably be like, "It's not mine. You'd best talk
to somebody else." I ended up telling him first, and it
wasn't as hard as I thought it would be. He didn't
seem mad, he seemed more surprised and confused.*

LaTisha, pregnant at 15

The longer you wait, the fewer options you have available. If you aren't pregnant, and you continue unprotected
sex, you're likely to *become* pregnant. In addition, fear of
pregnancy is scary and extremely stressful. Don't prolong
the agony of wondering if you're pregnant or not.

Do You Think You're Pregnant?

*I thought I might be pregnant a long time before I
saw the doctor. I was six months along before I went.*

Terry, pregnant at 16

If you think you are, then chances are you're right. If you're not sure, it's important to find out right away.

Pregnant women need special medical attention. Most pregnancies go along normally, but usually the woman needs to take care with her diet. She needs to make sure she's not doing anything that might harm her baby.

Please do one or more of the following *immediately*:

- **Contact a local women's center or clinic.**
  You can find these clinics or centers through the local Yellow Pages under "Birth Control Information Centers." Be aware that some clinics, especially those listed under "alternatives," do not perform abortions. If you don't want to eliminate abortion as a choice, select another doctor or clinic.

- **Talk to your school counselor.**
  If you feel you can talk to a teacher or school counselor more easily than to a family member or a stranger, please see one immediately. S/he will probably direct you to the best place to get help.

- **Buy a home pregnancy test.**
  Do you feel confident that you can take a home pregnancy test, accurately follow the directions, and read the results? If so, go to the nearest drug store and buy the kit (in the personal hygiene area), usually for under fifteen dollars. If done correctly, these tests are accurate.
  A positive result always means you're pregnant. However, a negative result does not necessarily let you off the hook. If you test negative and continue having symptoms, retake the test a week later, or go to a clinic to be checked.

- **Tell your mother, family member, or other adult friend.**
  If you have an open relationship with your parent or an adult friend, it's probably best to tell her/him about your problem first. I don't recommend this, however, if you're afraid of revealing your pregnancy. If that's the case, you're likely to put off telling that person until you can no longer hide your pregnancy.

  In addition, if that person has strong opinions on what pregnant girls should do, such as having or not having an abortion, s/he could add to your confusion if you consider another choice.

- **Tell your baby's father (if he doesn't already know).**
  If he doesn't know already, he will probably find out. He may offer support or advice or just another opinion. If he is abusive or unconcerned, don't try to "turn him around." You'll need your energy to take control of your life.

Let's Discuss Your Options

After you find out for sure that you're pregnant, don't panic. It happens to teens every day and in every community. You'll find there are many people prepared to help you. Your options are:

- Have an abortion.

- Have the baby and place it for adoption.

- Have the baby and parent him/her (with or without the father).

We'll talk more about these three options later. Just be assured that you *will* be able to make the choice that is right for you.

What Is *Not* an Option?

Do you have so many ideas about what to do that you're confused? Some of these ideas may be good, some bad. Thinking about them allows you to consider all your options.

You need help dealing with your situation. Some of the options you might consider could be damaging to you and add to your problems.

These things are *not* options:

- **Trying to bring on miscarriage**

  Too hot or too cold baths, starving yourself, jumping off anything, falling downstairs, or taking various home remedies may hurt you or make you sick. In fact, these techniques generally leave you pregnant *and* sick or injured.

  Also keep in mind that later you may decide to have the baby. If you take any drugs or chemicals in early pregnancy, they could harm the baby.

- **Suicide**

  This is not only an end to a pregnancy, but to your life as well. This problem can be faced and dealt with. Death is final. Suicide is a permanent solution to a temporary problem. What should you do if you're seriously considering suicide? Ask for help immediately.

  Even if you don't feel like talking to someone you know, call a Suicide Crisis line. Don't choose someone who you know might make you feel worse.

  For instance, don't try to confront your boyfriend if you're upset about a break-up. After this crisis has passed, be absolutely sure you ask for counseling.

- **Running away**
  It may seem easier to run away and try to make it on your own rather than facing your parent's anger and hurt. You need emotional and medical support right now. Running away will cause a whole new set of problems.

- **Relying on people who are not helping you**
  Sometimes a boyfriend or girlfriend will try to "help" you by talking you into things that will only prolong your problem or make it worse. For example, someone might tell you not to do anything because you might miscarry or have your period. Someone might even offer to help you get rid of the pregnancy. Advice like this can only add to your problems.

Getting Medical Help

Once you reveal your pregnancy to a responsible adult or clinic, they will make sure that you get the medical care you need right now.

WARNING: If that responsible adult or friend is not steering you in the direction of help, you have not yet talked to the right person. If your mother or friend is unable to reveal your pregnancy to an outside clinic or doctor, you have not yet gotten the help you need. Try another option.

It is important that you read as much as you can about pregnancy and the medical and emotional symptoms. This is important so that you know what your body needs right now in order to stay healthy.

An excellent prenatal health book written especially for pregnant teens is *Teens Parenting—Your Pregnancy and*

Newborn Journey by Jeanne Lindsay and Jean Brunelli
(1994: Morning Glory Press).

Getting Emotional Help

It is just as important for you to get emotional help and
support as it is to get medical support. Your emotional
health can affect your medical health. That's why you may
get sick when you're stressed out about something. A good
clinic has counselors who will help you untangle your
feelings.

There are other things you can do. You can join a support group. (Find one through the clinic or through your
high school counselor.) You can read all you can find on
pregnancy and how it affects your emotions. Public
libraries carry such books or can get them for you.

Most importantly, *you* can control your own health by
making your own decisions and keeping control of your
situation.

Other Problems

Most of us have different kinds of problems, some of
them minor and some major. Lots of teenagers deal every
day with more serious problems. Some may even see
pregnancy as a "way out." Do you have any of these
compounding problems?

Abuse

Unfortunately, many teenagers live with abuse (sexual,
emotional, and physical). As much as people don't like to
think about it, pregnancies sometimes result from sexual
abuse.

Emotional and physical abuse (beatings, pushing and
shoving, physical threats) can compound your pregnancy
problem because you may feel that you're alone.

You certainly cannot count on help from someone who abuses you.

You need someone to trust and in whom you can confide. Go to a teacher, counselor, clinic, or other trusted adult. Be sure to talk not only about your pregnancy, but also about your abuse and other problems.

Are You a Runaway?

Each year, more than two million teens run away from home. If you're one of them, you're probably running away from something, not toward something better. You may have run away out of fear of facing parents (and others) about your pregnancy. You may have additional problems in your home such as abuse or violence.

If you can't call home, there are places to go for help. They understand what you're going through, and they won't just tell you to "go home." Most cities have local shelters for runaway teens.

There are maternity homes for pregnant teens. You may hear about one from other teens. If you don't, you could go to a local clinic and ask for help. You could call the telephone operator and ask her to look up telephone numbers for you.

Drug Use/Dependency

About one third of high school seniors have used illegal drugs at some time, according to *The New Teenage Body Book Guide* by Kathy McCoy and Charles Wibbelsman, M.D. (1992: Putnam Publishing Group). The most common is alcohol. Cocaine and crack, PCP, amphetamines and barbiturates, heroin, LSD, marijuana, and tobacco are also used.

Some teens say they use drugs to cope with shyness, nervousness, loneliness, anger or social awkwardness. You may think you need drugs to help you deal with family problems, poverty, or other situations over which you feel no control.

Alcohol can cause problems for pregnant women. Fetal Alcohol Syndrome (FAS) is a disorder that is linked to drinking during pregnancy. These babies may be mentally retarded and have heart, face, and body defects. The National Council of Alcoholism and the March of Dimes Birth Defects Foundation recommend that pregnant women stay away from liquor altogether during pregnancy. (I shudder when I think of the bottle of gin I shared with my friend that night many years ago when I desperately wanted not to be pregnant. What a terrible risk!)

Smoking can cause smaller-than-normal babies, and has been linked to miscarriage. Be sure to tell your doctor or clinic if you smoke. If you plan to continue your pregnancy, stop smoking immediately if you possibly can. If you can't stop, can you cut back on your cigarettes? Your baby would appreciate you.

Heroin, cocaine, and crack can cause HIV infection leading to AIDS (from injecting drugs) and death. In addition, a pregnant woman can pass an addiction through the placenta to her unborn child.

Prescription drugs (drugs that your doctor has given to you) should be stopped immediately when you suspect that you're pregnant. Tetracycline (an antibiotic) can stain the baby's teeth, Accutane (sometimes given to treat acne) can cause birth defects.

In addition, there are many other examples of drugs you should not take when you're pregnant. If you have a special health problem, such as diabetes, it is critical that you see a doctor *immediately*.

There is no easy answer to drug addiction. If you even think you *might* have this problem, don't be afraid to tell your counselor or doctor. They need to know to help you.

The New Teenage Body Book lists these ways of helping yourself with a drug problem:

1) Stop your habit "just for today." Don't say, "I will never again pick up a cigarette." Sometimes forever is a promise you cannot keep.

2) Take responsibility for your choices.

3) Don't put yourself in situations where the pressure is great.

4) Learn from the pressure. Peer pressure can be a learning experience. If you can withstand the pressure and make your own choices, you'll have a good start toward healthy adulthood.

5) Announce your intentions to your family and friends.

6) Find the best way of stopping—for you.

7) Seek healthy alternatives and be patient with yourself.

What Will Happen to You?

Once you get help, things will happen fast. Your family will find out. This sounds bad, but it's really good. It means that things are happening, you can start talking and moving forward—and making decisions.

You must start understanding what has happened to you and why. You probably understand to some extent the biological, physical reason you got pregnant. In addition, you need to understand yourself and your motives because this will help you make the decision that is most right for you.

You may be afraid your parents will kick you out, or worse. In reality, most parents care enough about their children to worry for their health and safety. Few young women find themselves homeless because of pregnancy.

Through the years, as I was raising my daughter, I often encountered discouraging statistics and comments on the odds of overcoming a teenage pregnancy. I heard so many times that "your life is ruined" that I began to think about what that statement means.

It's hard to ruin a life. The only thing that ruins life is not living. I believe that anyone can overcome any kind of odds if she is determined and truly believes she can—and if she gets the help she needs.

That's not to say that it's easy. It's not. There are no easy solutions to too-early pregnancy. The remaining chapters will guide you on decision-making, and encourage you to make the most of the rest of your life.

Your life is not over!

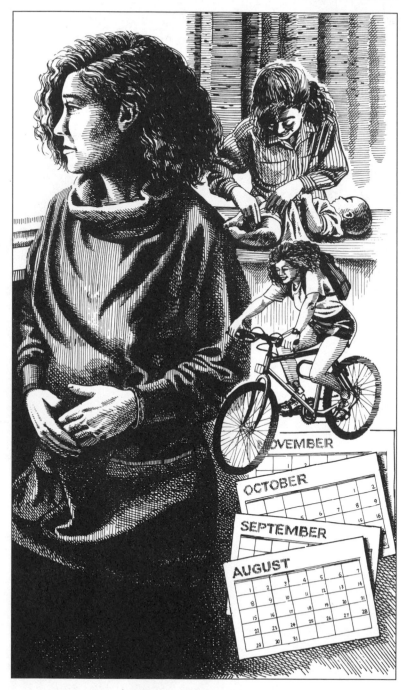

CHAPTER 2

YOU ARE
NOT ALONE

.

> Not to me—always to someone else,
> as one naturally thinks of disaster.
> Not to me—always to someone else,
> as one thinks also of the most wanted.
> Margaret Laurence—Rachel, Rachel

Carol's Story

*Carol was 13 years old and she lived in a poor
neighborhood. She lived with her mother, a sister, and two
brothers. Her mother worked long, hard hours to support
the family. Carol and her sister shared many responsibilities in caring for the house and their two younger
brothers while their mother made a living for them.*

*Carol met John, who lived in their apartment building.
John was 17, a basketball player with dreams of being a*

*professional player. He had a potential scholarship to a
state university. To Carol, he seemed like a way out. She
fell in love with him.*

*John, unlike a lot of other boys she knew, didn't smoke,
drink, or use drugs. He was dedicated to basketball and
his future.*

*John treated Carol like she was something special, and
they began having sex almost immediately. Carol was
excited at the new sensations of being loved, touched, and
held. It was magical for her. She felt loved and special for
the first time in her life. She quickly did her work every day
after school so that her sister could take over and she could
see John.*

"It's better than the way I live now.
So what if we have a baby?
We love each other."

---

*Carol knew she could get pregnant. Her older sister had
warned her many times, but Carol didn't care. "It's better
than the way I live now," she thought. "So what if we have
a baby? We love each other. The baby and I would go away
with him while he goes to school. I'd take care of the house
and baby the same as I do now for Mom."*

*Carol missed a period almost immediately and knew she
was pregnant. She was sick in the morning and tired all the
time. She told her sister, who was upset about it and didn't
want to tell their mom.*

*Carol told John, who got scared. He and his mother
moved away. They didn't bother to tell Carol where
they went.*

*Carol was sure that John would return when he was
successful. She decided to have the baby and keep it so
their family would remain intact.*

Michelle, the Last Girl
Anyone Thought Would Get Pregnant

Michelle was 16, an honor student, and extremely shy. She was never especially popular, and she always felt like an outsider, like a spectator of life but never a player. Her friends told her she was pretty. They said nobody ever noticed because of her shyness.

A year ago, Michelle met Todd. Todd was attractive and a little on the wild side. Michelle's parents didn't approve of him which bothered Michelle a little, but her attraction to Todd was strong. Todd knew lots of people and took her to all the parties. Everybody knew Todd, and Michelle wanted them to know her, too. She began drinking because everybody drank at the parties.

Soon after their relationship started, Todd began pressuring Michelle about sex. She liked being held and caressed, and she began having physical urges to have sex. The thought of sex frightened her a little because she knew she could get pregnant. She knew about birth control, too, but the thought of going to the doctor and asking for pills terrified her. He would know that she was having sex, and besides, he might tell her parents.

Her mother always told Michelle to come to her if she needed birth control, but Michelle was too scared to do that. What if her mom made her break up with Todd?

He found condoms a pain to use.
"It feels much better without," he told her.

Michelle quit talking to most of her friends. She was always with Todd, and she didn't seem to need them anymore. She gave in to Todd's advances, and once they started having sex, they continued. Todd used condoms a couple of times during the middle of Michelle's cycle, but he found them a pain to use. "It feels much better without," he told her.

Michelle took a pack of her mom's birth control pills from her dresser and took them all at once, thinking that they would make her temporarily infertile. Then she decided not to worry about pregnancy.

About five months later, Todd began treating Michelle differently. He was verbally mean to her in front of other people. He teased her about being shy, and that hurt her deeply.

After that, Michelle saw him only occasionally. They never really broke up, so Michelle waited for him to come around to party with her. Her grades dropped. Her periods stopped and she lost weight, but she was sure this was due to stress. She felt she could even be infertile and never able to have children. She decided to wait and not worry about anything but getting Todd back.

Kim, Too

Kim, a mature high school junior, met John at a party. John was everything Kim ever wanted, and she was totally in love. The only problem was that John was 28 and she was only 16. She couldn't wait until she was 18 and could leave home. John promised her that he would take care of her, and he had enough money to take her places and buy her things.

Since John was so much older, he expected sex right away. Kim knew that he had many other girlfriends in the past, and she didn't want to lose him. Besides, he would take care of her if anything happened.

John used condoms a few times, but several times they didn't. After a few months, Kim realized that she was pregnant. She told John, and he became angry, telling her that he didn't need to be tied down. He began dating other young women. Kim's parents were supportive, and helped Kim get child support from John.

The Same Problem

Carol, Michelle, and Kim have the same problem. They are all teenagers, and they are all pregnant.

They are all frightened and confused. Yet, they are different. Each has unique circumstances. Their stories are different, but the result—pregnancy—is the same.

What Are You Feeling?

When we have a problem that hurts us or scares us, we go through several emotional stages. These stages help us deal with things gradually, when we're ready. Teenage pregnant girls often go through the same emotions, though not always in the same order.

Remember, too, that each girl's situation may be a little different depending on how much support she gets from her boyfriend, family, friends, and others. One young woman might be happy about her pregnancy, and another might be devastated.

When I realized I was pregnant, I was happy. Of course our parents were upset, and we had to go through all that. I was happy because I felt it was giving me something to fill my life.

Cathi, pregnant at 16

While I was pregnant, I was confused and depressed. I didn't like being pregnant. It was an awful experience for me. Just because I felt so fat, I thought my boyfriend didn't want to be with me. I thought he was there only because he felt sorry for me.

Frederica, pregnant at 15

You might feel some of these emotions:

Shock

You probably knew you could get pregnant, but you didn't think you *would*. Sometimes shock feels like an electrical shock that shoots through us, numbing our feelings when we hear something we're not ready to hear. This is the "auto accidents happen to other people" feeling that keeps you from worrying all the time about what *could* happen. Then, if it does happen, you don't believe it, or you think it'll just go away.

Shock has the important job of protecting us from knowing something that we are not yet ready to know. This leads to denial.

Denial

Some young women go out of their way to avoid finding out they're pregnant. They make excuses to themselves about why they don't have periods, why they're sick every morning, and even why they feel "fluttering" in their stomach. Young women do this when the thought of pregnancy is more than the mind can handle. Some girls convince themselves that they are infertile, that they have the flu or some other illness.

Seventeen-year-old Sharon lived with her boyfriend for a year before she got pregnant, but she still couldn't believe it:

> *I kind of knew I was pregnant, but when the doctor told me I was five months, I told him there was no way. You know it, but you don't want to deal with it. You push it to the back of your mind.*

Denial is dangerous because some girls never accept their pregnancy. They don't get the medical care they need, and some end up delivering their babies alone. Obviously, you are not one of those girls, or you would not be reading this book.

You may drift in and out of denial though, and sometimes we need to do this to cope with a teen pregnancy. When we do confront our pregnancy, we often experience some fear.

Fear

I was more scared than I've ever been in my life.
So was he.

Donna, pregnant at 17

Fear is a common reaction. You may not have realized what it means to be pregnant. You may even have fantasized about being pregnant and sharing something with your boyfriend. You may have been fearful about becoming pregnant, but didn't think it would happen to you. Your fear may have made you deny your condition until your pregnancy was advanced. The best relief for fear is to tell someone who can help you.

Loneliness

While I hope that you have someone to talk to, many girls do not, or are too shy to tell anyone about their pregnancy. Loneliness causes depression and may lead to an unhealthy escape from reality. Even if you confide in one or more people, you may continue to feel lonely and scared.

Anger

At some point during your pregnancy, you're likely to be angry. You may be angry with your parents, boyfriend, friends, even teachers. You may be angry with yourself for becoming pregnant.

Many teens feel angry with their boyfriends for deserting them or for not coming up with a magical solution to the problem. The fact is that your parents, friends, and

boyfriend may not know how to handle this problem any
better than you do. They may be angry with you for "letting
this happen" or for disrupting their lives. Some young
women feel anger toward the baby they are carrying.

Depression

Depression and sadness are different things. Everyone
feels sad at times, but sometimes a problem like pregnancy
causes a deeper feeling of depression.

Many pregnant girls get depressed for good reasons:
their lives are turned upside down; their friends lose interest in them; their boyfriends drift away; they find themselves with big responsibilities.

You may feel like hiding in your room. You may not
feel like eating or sleeping.

Your parents may be depressed about your pregnancy,
too. They may see your pregnancy as a long-term financial
burden, and as more of a problem to them than to you.

The loss of a boyfriend can bring on severe depression.
Contrary to what many adults believe, teenage love can be
more intense than adult love. If you have broken up with
your boyfriend, you may feel abandoned and betrayed.

Distortion of Reality

Distorting reality sometimes helps us deal with difficult
truths. Wishing for miscarriage is one way to distort the
reality of a pregnancy. It happens all the time on television:
an inconvenient pregnancy ends in miscarriage, the woman
weeps, and it is all over.

Some girls distort reality by waiting for a boyfriend or
lover to rescue them. This seldom happens because he's
usually in no position to rescue anyone. Sometimes this
fantasy persists even when the boy has become involved
with someone else.

Apathy

Apathy is a "nothingness" or a feeling that you don't care. Disinterest in your pregnancy or its outcome is another way of taking yourself away from the trauma or the decisions you are not prepared to make. You may simply decide to do nothing or wait and see what happens.

This is slightly different from denial because this occurs after you have admitted your pregnancy to yourself and your family. They may be shocked that you continue to live your life as usual, as though nothing is wrong. Maybe you continue to go to local night-spots or out partying with your friends. Maybe you refuse to talk to anyone about making decisions, or what you plan for the future. This stage is not likely to last because the progress of the pregnancy will force you into a different stage.

Happiness and Hopefulness

It's not uncommon for a girl to be happy about a pregnancy. You may have wanted to get pregnant (for reasons we'll discuss later), and now you have feelings of happiness mixed in with other feelings.

I wanted to get pregnant, so I'm happy. I really love my boyfriend, so now we'll always have this baby together.

Lara, pregnant at 17

This feeling of happiness is common in girls who have plans to marry the baby's father, or feel this pregnancy will please him or someone else. There is a feeling of creativity that comes with being pregnant—as though you're building something wonderful.

Confusion

You will probably have a healthy mixture of all these emotions throughout your pregnancy. They come and go like the tide moving in and out. This causes confusion. You are tired and torn in many directions, and you may not feel capable of making decisions. You may want someone to take over and make them for you.

As parents, teachers, and boyfriends become aware of your pregnancy, you may become more confused because you will get all kinds of advice and will not know which to follow. Don't be surprised at changing emotions. You may go to bed one night anguished over your situation and wake up the next day feeling hopeful and happy.

How Pregnancy Affects Your Emotions

I thought I was happy about the pregnancy, but I went around crying all the time.

Sharon, pregnant at 16

Hormones are chemicals that your body produces to prepare it for nine months of pregnancy. These same hormones can cause wild mood swings, crying jags, and sickness. If you are throwing up every morning or all day long, obviously this is not doing much for your mental health. You may be tired and cranky.

These physical symptoms are made worse by depression and stress. A doctor may be able to give you tips on controlling morning sickness with diet and mental attitude. Taking the vitamins your doctor prescribes may help you feel less tired.

It is important not to self-treat, but to let the doctor do what s/he does best. The important thing to realize is that you probably are not going crazy. Some of the things you are experiencing are normal.

Good Nutrition

Eating right during your pregnancy will help you feel better and stronger. You'll be stronger for delivery and have a healthier baby. You don't really have to eat for two, but you do need to eat *better.* You make choices every time you eat. Candy bars, cakes, and soda pop don't have many nutrients, and they're high in calories. For snacks, you could have popcorn, fruit, vegetables, or cheese instead.

Do you have to give up fast food? Most teens like hamburgers, fries, and pizza. It's okay to have these sometimes. Pizza has meat, cheese, and bread, but it's not good to live on fast food. If you eat in a fast-food place, try the salad bar instead of a burger and fries.

Your doctor will probably give you vitamins, and it's important to take these every day. Try to drink 6 to 8 glasses of water a day. Exercising every day helps keep your energy up and aids in controlling your weight. Walking is a good form of exercise.

What Can You Do?

Find someone you can talk to. Nobody can make all of your problems disappear, but talking about your feelings can make them seem less threatening. If you can't talk to a friend or relative, find a teen pregnancy support group through your school or a nearby clinic.

Understanding that you are normal and that you are not alone will help you. Don't make any quick decisions when you're feeling emotional (angry, depressed, upset). Give yourself time to work out your emotions, talk to someone about how you feel, then *move on to decision making.*

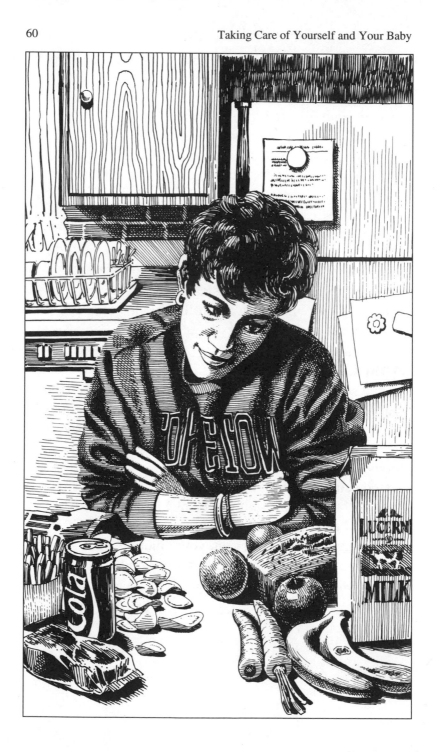

CHAPTER 3

TAKING CARE OF YOU AND YOUR BABY

Many teens wait until late in their pregnancy to see the doctor. This means that during the early months, they may not have eaten right or gotten the extra vitamins they need for a healthy pregnancy.

Special Needs of Teen Mothers

Very young mothers are at higher risk of having a premature baby with health problems. They also have a higher chance of having a baby with low birthweight. These babies sometimes take extra time and care to catch up with normal weight babies. Some young mothers are not aware that things they indulge in, like drinking alcohol and smoking or drug use, can harm their baby.

It's possible to have a serious problem with your pregnancy and not be aware of it. You wouldn't know if you had high blood pressure unless a doctor or nurse told you.

You also probably wouldn't know if you were anemic

(too little iron in your blood), or if the baby is lying in the correct position for childbirth. That's why seeing a doctor is so important.

You may still be growing yourself. If so, it's especially important to get all the vitamins and minerals you need to keep yourself and your baby healthy.

Nutrition

Your nutritional needs are at an all-time high when you're pregnant. What you eat affects your health and your baby's. Maybe you've heard that you need to "eat for two" now. You don't really need to eat much *more* food when you're pregnant, but you need to eat the right kinds of foods. Experts say that you need only an additional 300 to 400 calories per day when you're pregnant.

To get the nutrients you need while pregnant, you'll need to eat a variety of foods from the basic food groups. These are:

1) Grains, bread, and cereal (6 to 11 servings). A serving is 1/2 cup grain or cereal, or one slice of bread. This group includes pasta, rice, cereals, tortillas, and starchy vegetables such as potatoes.

2) Vegetables (3 to 5 servings). A serving is 1/2 cup fresh or cooked vegetables or 1 cup leafy greens. This group includes all fresh, frozen, or canned vegetables. Fresh is better, if possible.

3) Fruit (2 to 4 servings). One serving is an average-size fruit, or approximately 1/2 cup. This includes fruit juices.

4) Dairy products (3 to 4 servings). One serving is 1 cup milk or yogurt, or a slice of cheese.

5) Protein (3 servings). A serving is 2 to 3 ounces of

lean meat, chicken, or fish, 2 large eggs, 1 cup cooked beans, or 4 tablespoons peanut butter.

6) Fats and sweets. Only a small amount of fat and sugar should be eaten each day.

See the chart on the next page for examples.
Your body requires a steady supply of nutrients or "fuel" to keep it going. A few tips:

- Try not to skip meals. You don't really save any calories. You make up for it later.

- Eat a variety of foods. Some people like the comfort of eating the same foods all the time. Maybe you like pizza. That's okay because pizza has nutrients. But if you eat only pizza all the time you will miss some other important nutrients.

- Drink plenty of water. It helps with digestion and keeps your skin healthy and pretty.

- Take healthy snacks to work or school. Fruit, granola bars, nuts, or popcorn may keep you away from vending machine candy bars and chips.

- Natural foods are best. Processed lunch meats have lots of salt and chemicals in them. Fresh fruits and vegetables are better for you than canned.

How Much Should You Gain?

Your doctor will weigh you during each office visit. Most doctors recomend 28-40 pounds gain throughout your pregnancy. If you're in your early teens, you should gain a little more than you would if you were older because you're still growing yourself.

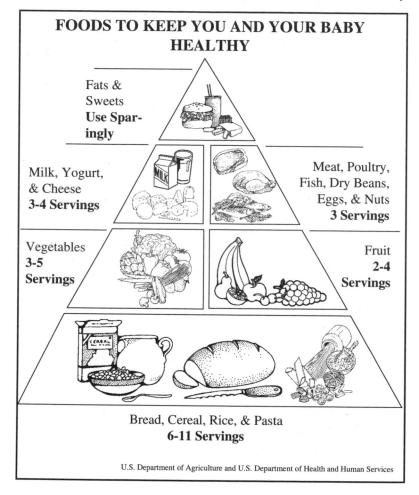

FOODS TO KEEP YOU AND YOUR BABY HEALTHY

Fats & Sweets
Use Sparingly

Milk, Yogurt, & Cheese
3-4 Servings

Meat, Poultry, Fish, Dry Beans, Eggs, & Nuts
3 Servings

Vegetables
3-5 Servings

Fruit
2-4 Servings

Bread, Cereal, Rice, & Pasta
6-11 Servings

U.S. Department of Agriculture and U.S. Department of Health and Human Services

The baby will normally weigh around seven pounds. The rest of your added weight is made up of extra water, extra blood, the placenta, your uterus, and an increase in your other body tissues.

Your doctor will alert you if you're gaining too much weight. Sometimes teen mothers don't gain enough weight. If you don't gain enough, your baby may not be getting enough nutrients. If the baby doesn't get enough nutrients, s/he may have health problems.

What about Junk Food?

Junk food isn't always "junk." Most of us like to indulge in fast-food hamburgers and fries sometimes. The trick is not to eat them all the time. Getting a good variety of foods is one way to make sure you get all the nutrients you need to keep healthy.

A fast-food cheeseburger has meat, grain (bun), and dairy (cheese). Fast food is usually high in calories, so if you're concerned about your weight, try to choose a smaller size hamburger or order pizza with vegetables instead of pepperoni.

You can make a fast-food meal more nutritious by having a milk shake instead of a soft drink, and by having a salad instead of french fries.

It helps to keep nutritious snacks around, like raw fruits and vegetables. If you don't keep chocolate chip cookies and potato chips around, you're less likely to eat them. Keeping lots of sweet and salty snacks in the house may encourage binging.

Exercise Helps

Exercise helps your body burn calories faster, helps build your immune system, and helps your mental attitude. It will help you keep your "shape" during and after your pregnancy.

Some medical experts think that exercise helps make childbirth easier. Walking is one of the best exercises for pregnant women—if they have a safe place to walk.

Prenatal exercise classes provide stretching and strength-building exercise for pregnant women. See if your local recreation center, health clinic, hospital, adult school, or high/junior high school sponsors such a class.

Some exercises may not be appropriate when you're pregnant, so consult your doctor first.

Smoking, Drinking, Drugs

If you smoke, drink alcohol, or use drugs, so does your baby. Whatever you put into your system passes through your blood stream into your baby's. It's best not to take any medication without asking your doctor first.

If you smoke, you might have a smaller baby, and he may not be as healthy as he could be. If you don't think you can stop smoking while you're pregnant, try to cut down.

Drinking when pregnant can cause Fetal Alcohol Syndrome. This can affect the baby's looks, her growth, and her brain. It's best not to drink alcohol at all while you're pregnant. As the March of Dimes Birth Defects Foundation points out, Fetal Alcohol Syndrome is the birth defect only the mother can prevent.

Preparing for Childbirth

Giving birth is hard work, and it's different for everybody. If you're prepared for what will happen during childbirth, you'll have an easier time.

Ask your doctor or teacher about childbirth preparation classes. They'll teach you about what happens during labor and delivery and how you can prepare yourself. Breathing exercises help give you control during labor and delivery, and most childbirth classes teach them.

Your Appearance

You'll notice a lot of changes while you're pregnant. Your complexion may get clearer and your nails stronger. Or, if you're not eating right, the opposite could happen. Sometimes the vitamins that doctors prescribe to pregnant women improve the hair, nails, and skin. It's a kind of bonus for being healthy.

Some changes you may not like. Some women get stretch marks on their stomach, legs, and breasts as they get

larger. There's not much you can do about this except keep
your skin soft with lotion or oil. It won't make the marks
go away, but your skin may become softer and less dry.

Clothes can affect how you feel about yourself. If you're
on a tight budget, you may worry about buying maternity
clothes. Some young women modify some of their regular
clothes to wear during pregnancy. Jeans can be modified
with a stretch panel. You can continue to wear stretch pants
and shorts, large sweaters, and T-shirts during much of
your pregnancy. Some men's shirts and T-shirts work well.

You don't need to shop at expensive maternity shops
because you can still wear stretch pants and baggy tops
after you deliver. You may be able to swap maternity
clothes with other young women, or find a second-hand
store that specializes in maternity fashions.

Taking Care of Yourself

You may be worried and upset about your pregnancy,
and that makes it harder to think about taking care of
yourself and eating right. You don't need the additional
problems of illness, pregnancy complications, or a sick or
unhealthy baby.

Even small things help like drinking a glass of milk
when you think of it, taking a walk when you need an
energy boost, or passing up a cigarette when you feel like
smoking. *Your baby will appreciate your efforts.*

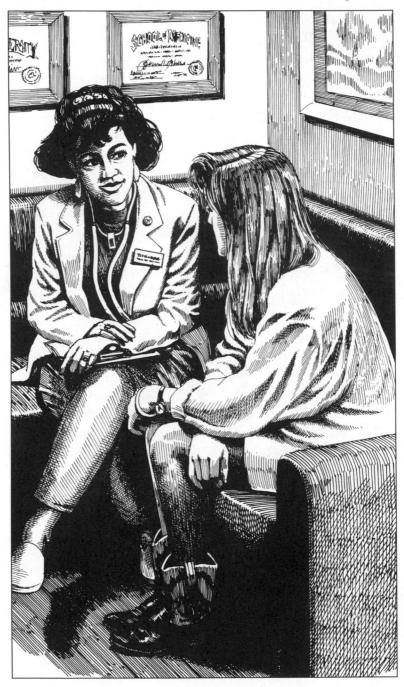

Introduction

MAKING CHOICES

I saw my life branching out before me
like the green fig tree . . .
From the tip of every branch, like a fat purple fig,
a wonderful future beckoned and winked.
I saw myself sitting in the crotch of this fig tree,
starving to death,
just because I couldn't make up my mind
which of the figs I would choose.

Sylvia Plath—*The Bell Jar*

The next three chapters talk about choices. The order of the chapters does not mean that one choice is better than another, or that one is more "right" than another. How to make your decision once you know about the alternatives is discussed in chapter 7.

You're probably already aware of your options. You're probably also aware of the arguments surrounding the abortion alternative. At this point in time, abortion is an option for pregnant women. I suspect that for most of you reading this book, however, abortion is not a choice. You may be too far along in your pregnancy, or you may have already ruled out this option.

Making decisions is one of the privileges of being an adult. It's also confusing because we usually want to know that we're making the *right* choice. It's hard to be sure.

It almost feels like the old shell game where a coin is hidden under a shell and you have to guess which one. *Sometimes, more than one shell has a coin under it.*

CHAPTER 4

ABORTION— A DIFFICULT CHOICE

Abortion means ending the pregnancy. You may know that abortion is a controversial choice, and you probably have heard about abortion protests.

More than a third of pregnant teenagers choose this option. However, many teenagers don't recognize their pregnancy until after the first three months when abortion may no longer be an option.

In most states, it's possible to get an abortion. The decision to have an abortion may not be easy, but it is still a legal option. Many people have strong beliefs that ending a pregnancy is ending a life, and for those people, abortion is wrong. Others believe differently.

Women have always had abortions and probably always will. Now that abortion is legal, women can obtain safe, medically supervised abortions. Most abortions are done during the first trimester of pregnancy (first three months) and are medically safe and relatively pain-free.

Statistics show that abortion is up to nine times safer than childbirth. For teens this is especially true. Teens have a 60 percent higher death rate for pregnancy and childbirth than older mothers, but they have the lowest abortion death rate.

A good clinic will give you psychological care, medical care, and birth control counseling. Just because you chose the best option for you doesn't mean it was an easy decision to make. You need (and deserve) good counseling.

You may be more confused about what you want. If you think you *might* want an abortion, or you're not sure, or your friends or family are pushing you one way or another, I strongly urge you to get counseling.

What Is Abortion?

Abortion means removing the growing fetus and placenta from the uterus. After an abortion, you are no longer pregnant.

How Is It Done?

Vacuum aspiration is used in 75 percent of first-trimester abortions. It's just the way it sounds: a small tube connected to a suction device is inserted through the cervix (opening to the uterus), and the contents of the uterus are suctioned out.

Dilatation and Currettage (D and C) is another method. Under local or general anesthesia, the cervix is dilated and the lining of the uterus is scraped to remove the contents.

Second-trimester (months three to five) abortions are more serious and complicated. A saline (salt) or prostaglandin (hormone) solution is injected into the uterus, replacing the amniotic fluid. This causes contractions, and the fetus is then expelled within 24 hours. Sometimes the D and C procedure is used on second trimester pregnancies.

Many states have laws setting time limits for these abortions, such as 24 weeks of pregnancy. Abortions during the thirteenth to twenty-fourth week of pregnancy may be called "gray-area" abortions. The pregnancy is in that gray area where a simple abortion is no longer possible because the fetus is too big. Many doctors have strong moral feelings against doing abortions during the second trimester.

Abortions are not performed after the twenty-fourth week of pregnancy because after that time the baby is fully formed and capable of living outside the womb.

What Does It Cost?

Changing abortion laws affect the cost of abortion, and the cost can vary from state to state. Costs also change because of differences in government funding of abortions. A clinic will let you know what the cost is when you call.

Some states provide financial help to low income women wanting abortions. Some health insurance covers abortions. Second-trimester abortions are a more serious procedure and are double or triple the cost of first-trimester abortions.

Is It Painful?

First-trimester abortion (whether a D and C or suction) is described as anywhere between almost painless and moderately painful. The procedure takes about ten minutes. Usually a local anesthesia is given to numb the vaginal-cervical area.

Some clinics give general anesthesia, but risks are greater because you are put to sleep with medication, and that's always more risky. The stay at the clinic or hospital is approximately an hour longer.

With a clinic abortion, you will be home the same day. You may have menstrual-like cramps and bleeding for a week or two, and you will be advised to watch for fever and excessive bleeding.

Second-trimester abortions take longer and are more painful. This is because you are going through labor to expel the fetus.

Some medication can be given, but not enough to take away all the pain since that would stop the labor and prolong the process.

Bleeding and cramping are common after this type of abortion. Some women even produce milk in their breasts. Recovery may be similar to recovery after childbirth.

Will You Be Depressed—Or Worse?

This may depend on whether or not you get adequate counseling before and after your decision. If you are talked into an abortion that you do not want, you may try to replace your loss later with another pregnancy.

If the decision is yours, and you are sure that's what you want, you'll probably be okay with some counseling. We are all unique emotionally as well as physically. It's impossible to say that "most" women either do or don't have problems after abortion.

> *I think I did the right thing but it's so hard. I still have to hear it every day at school. You don't want to sit there and cry. There were a few friends that were supportive.*
>
> Raylene, pregnant at 15

Some women have post-abortion depression. This may be related to hormone shifts, although some feeling of loss can be expected. It is common to feel a little weepy for a while after the abortion. If the depression lasts for a long period of time (longer than two weeks), you need further

medical care or counseling. Most clinics provide counseling, but you may need to ask about it.

Where Should You Go
If You Want an Abortion?

Although hospitals and clinics were permitted to perform
abortions by 1973, they are not required to do so. Many
helping agencies will counsel against abortion, especially
those run by right-to-life groups or religious agencies. Not
all religious agencies, however, counsel against abortion.

You can check under "abortion" in the local Yellow
Pages. The listings under "abortion alternatives" or "alternatives" are likely to steer you away from abortion.

Will They Tell Anyone?

Abortion laws change all the time. Individual states now
have more freedom to pass laws on abortion. Some states
have more restrictions on abortion than others. Some states
have notification laws where the parents must be notified if
their teenager wants an abortion. Check with a local counselor, clinic, or the local Board of Health. They will have
up-to-date information.

If you decide on abortion, you'll need someone's support. A friend, a boyfriend, or a trusted relative can provide
you with emotional support and help before and after the
abortion.

*Jeff and I talked about it, and we went to the clinic
and they talked to us. He was with me.*

*Sometimes I'm in the mood, and I want to talk and
wonder if I made the right decision. It helps to talk
to him.*

Raylene

Please at least try to tell your parents. You may find that

they agree with your decision, and they can help you
financially and emotionally.

If you're sure you want an abortion, you should look
into it immediately. Your situation will not improve, and
you will be deciding by default to have a baby if you wait.
Most important, do not endanger your life by trying to
obtain an illegal abortion.

Risks and Side Effects

Having a safe abortion does not decrease your chances
of getting pregnant in the future, according to Robert Blum,
M.D., Obstetrician/Gynecologist, Kaiser Permanente,
Downey, California.

An infection can cause scarring of your reproductive
organs if left untreated. However, you will show signs such
as fever and pain if you have an infection, and it can be
promptly treated. This can happen with any infection, not
just those caused by abortion.

Nor do most girls have terrible nightmares, go crazy
with guilt, or attempt suicide after abortion (unless they
have serious emotional problems anyway, or have not
resolved their decision).

Abortions obtained from a safe, legal clinic are relatively risk-free. This doesn't mean it's easy or that you
won't need emotional help if you choose this option.
Choosing to stay pregnant isn't easy either. To repeat, it is
important to get good before and after counseling.

Pros and Cons

Reasons in favor of abortion:

- You feel you are too young to handle the responsibility of a baby, have little support from family
  members, and you know you can't follow through
  on an adoption.

- Your parents may not have to know that you were pregnant, although it's usually a good idea to tell them anyway.

- You and your family cannot handle the emotional or financial responsibility of another child, and you feel unable to place the baby with an adoptive family. You have agreed, and feel that the best option is abortion.

- You don't want this baby and don't feel you can provide it with a good life. You don't feel capable of placing the baby with another family.

Abortion is the wrong choice when:

- You have strong religious or personal beliefs against abortion.

- Your parents or boyfriend are pressuring you to have an abortion, and you do not want one.

- You're afraid to tell your parents or others about the pregnancy, and that's why you've decided to have an abortion.

Questions to Ask Yourself

The following questions should help you think about why you do or do not want an abortion. Remember that if you get an abortion, it should be because you believe that it is right for you at this time. This is important to your future.

Studies show that girls who get abortions and feel regret over their decision become pregnant a second (or third) time. They may be a little older and feel they can better handle a baby (when in reality a couple of years doesn't make that much difference), or they subconsciously want to replace the lost baby.

Think about these questions:

- Does my boyfriend want this abortion and I don't? Does he promise a continued relationship if I abort the baby?

- Are my parents against the abortion and I'm not?

- Do I want an abortion only so my parents won't find out?

- Do I think I'll be upset after the abortion?

- Do I think abortion is wrong?

- Do I fantasize about this baby? In other words, do I fantasize about what he or she looks like, acts like, smells like, etc.?

- Do I think I deserve to be punished and believe that abortion is a punishment?

- Am I afraid to tell my parents that I'm pregnant?

Answering yes to any of these questions means that you need to think about your options further. It does not mean that you will be turned down for an abortion, or that abortion is not an option for you.

It could mean that you have some unresolved feelings of guilt, or you might suffer continuing emotional damage or repeated "surprise" pregnancies if you terminate this one.

On the other hand, if you know for certain that you want an abortion, if you get good before and after abortion counseling, and if you are within the first trimester of your pregnancy, you should have little or no problem coping with your decision.

Is It Too Late for This Option?

Teenage women are less likely than older women to recognize and admit their pregnancies promptly. You may even be in the final three months of your pregnancy when abortion is absolutely not an option. Only a physician or other medical person can guide you.

More than likely if your pregnancy is advanced, your options diminish to adoption or keeping the baby. Some young women see this as punishment or cruelty on the part of the doctor, but s/he is protecting you (and the baby) from further harm. If you are in the gray area that we talked about and are strongly motivated to have an abortion, you must talk to your doctor about that possibility. If s/he is unwilling to help you, try another clinic or doctor, or rethink your decision.

The very young, the very poor, and girls in rural areas are more likely to wait too long to obtain wanted abortions. This is either because of denial, lack of money, or lack of knowledge of where to go for help.

If it is truly too late to choose abortion, the best thing to do is try (with outside help) to come to grips with what is happening to you. Now you must make the best alternative choice for yourself and your child.

If you haven't already done so, tell your parents or someone else you trust about your pregnancy immediately. You need medical care and assistance *now*.

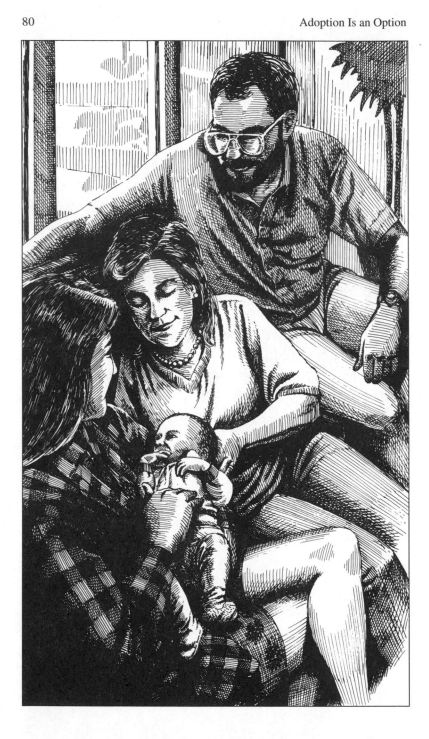

CHAPTER 5

ADOPTION
IS AN OPTION

Your children are not your children.
They are the sons and daughters of Life's longing
for itself.
They come through you but not from you,
And though they are with you, yet they belong not
to you.
You may give them your love but not your thoughts.
For they have their own thoughts.
You may house their bodies but not their souls,
For their souls dwell in the house of tomorrow,
which you cannot visit,
Not even in your dreams.
You may strive to be like them, but seek not to make
them like you.
For life goes not backward nor tarries with yesterday.

You are the bows from which your children as
living arrows are sent forth.

Kahlil Gibran—*The Prophet*

Years ago, most pregnant teenagers chose adoption.
Young and single pregnant women were expected to go
away, perhaps to a shelter for pregnant teenagers, place
their children for adoption, and then go on with their lives.
Usually it wasn't talked about again, and the young woman
probably received no counseling.

Now, fewer than four percent of unmarried pregnant
teens place their babies for adoption. This change is a result
of changing opinions about teen pregnancy.

Today, you may be discouraged by friends and family
from making an adoption plan. They may think that planning to adopt is "giving your baby away." You may think
that adoption might be the right answer, and maybe you're
afraid to admit it to friends or family.

I didn't find out I was pregnant until I was five
months. I decided right away that I probably wouldn't
keep him. I knew adoption would be better for him
and better for me.

My grandma thought adoption was unheard of, and
it was a real shock to her. I care about her, but I'm
glad I didn't change my mind because of her. My
mom was also against adoption. She would say, "I
raised you by myself, you can do it, too."

And I would say, "Look at what I went through. I
don't want that for him."

Nancy, pregnant at 17

Adoption is a giving, caring option. It doesn't mean that
you don't love your baby, or that you're abandoning him. It
means that you care enough to give him a good home when

you know you can't do that yourself.

More older teenagers and adult women consider adoption than young teenagers. Why is this?

Many teenage parents agree that it's hard to parent a child. It's hard to give him everything he needs to grow and develop as he should. On the other hand, many *pregnant* teens don't understand how difficult parenting is. Rather than considering these realities, some young women (and their partners) simply assume everything will work out okay when they become parents. They don't consider the adoption option.

If you're considering adoption today, you have more options than were available in the past.

Closed Adoption

Some adoptions are "closed." In a closed adoption, the birthmother might see the baby for an hour or two and then sign the adoption papers. A closed adoption means that you sign the papers releasing your baby without knowing the identity of his new family. You probably won't have any future contact with your child. Some young mothers want the confidentiality this option provides.

The baby may be released directly to the adoption agency rather than to the adoptive parents. In agency adoptions, the agency handles the details of the adoption. The records are sealed, and the revised birth certificate has only the name of the adoptive parents on it. There is no contact between the birthparents and adoptive parents, or between the birthparents and the child.

The birthparents, however, can usually write a letter to their baby. The letter would be given to the adoptive parents and the baby by a counselor or social worker. You might want to write a letter because you want your baby to know that you didn't just "give her away." *Did My First*

Mother Love Me? by Kathryn Miller (1994: Morning Glory Press) provides an example of such a letter as the major part of the story in this picture book for adoptees.

Open Adoption

In many cases today, however, all the people involved want more from adoption. Many grown adopted children are now searching for their birthparents. The adoptee may have a natural curiosity about her birthmother.

The birthmother may need to know about her child. She may need to know that her child is safe and healthy and receiving good care.

Birthparents and adoptive parents may want to share health information or other information about their child. They may want to continue seeing each other after the adoption is finalized. Open adoption gives you more choices and more control over your baby's life.

Open adoption can mean different things. You may be able to meet and choose the adoptive parents. You decide whether or not to make an adoption plan after you meet them. Or you may choose the adoptive parents from resumes which may contain their photograph and lots of information about them.

In some open adoptions, the child knows his birthparents. It doesn't mean that you'd parent the child together, but that you could visit the child if everyone involved agreed.

In the beginning, I visited my baby and his adoptive parents each week. It was hard seeing him with them even though that was my intention the whole time. I think he was meant to be with Carl and Louise. I was sure from the minute I met them.

Nancy

Adoptive parents must deal with their own feelings about the adoption. Since they usually cannot become pregnant, or have been pregnant and lost the baby, they may feel pain and grief. They may fear that the birthparents will change their minds about adoption. Sometimes meeting with or writing to the birthparents helps them, too.

Open adoption can help the birthparents and the adoptive parents feel more secure about their decision. The birthparents know that the baby is healthy and loved, and the adoptive parents understand the feelings of the birthparents. They are usually less likely to fear that the birthparents will change their minds and decide to parent their child themselves. Counseling helps the birthparents and adoptive parents understand their own and each other's feelings.

For more information about open adoption, see *Open Adoption: A Caring Option* (1987: Morning Glory Press).

Choosing An Agency

There are different kinds of adoption agencies. Each state has an agency that deals with adoption. This agency is probably called the Bureau of Family and Children's Services, the Division of Social Services, or the Department of Public Welfare. Cities and/or counties may have their own agencies. These can be found in the government listings of the telephone book. Some of these agencies may offer only closed adoptions.

Most states have licensed private adoption agencies. Some are associated with a certain religion or plan adoptions for children with special needs such as handicapped or minority children. Some agencies specialize in infant adoption and others specialize in adoption of older children.

More agencies are offering open adoptions although some still provide only closed placements. If you're

considering adoption, call a few local agencies and ask
them about open adoption.

You don't have to stick with the first agency or independent adoption service you contact. It may appear to be a
lot of trouble to shop around for the right agency, but it's
worth it for your peace of mind. If you don't feel comfortable, you feel like you're being pressured, or you don't get
adequate counseling, try another agency or independent
adoption service.

Independent Adoption

Independent adoption means going through a private
organization, doctor, or lawyer instead of an adoption
agency. The birthparents present the child directly to the
adoptive parents instead of to the adoption agency. Private
adoptions often allow the birthparents to choose the adoptive parents. In some cases, they allow for future contact
with the child.

A disadvantage to independent adoption is that the
birthmother is less likely to get counseling after the adoption. However, more and more across the country, independent adoption centers are providing counseling for
their clients.

In independent adoption, how do the birthparents and
adoptive parents find each other? There is a large network
of people interested in adopting babies. You may hear
about a reputable lawyer or doctor from a counselor or
from a friend or acquaintance who adopted a child. The
Yellow Pages list adoption resources.

You'll need more information if you're considering
independent adoption. You need to make sure the lawyer or
doctor you're dealing with is honest and has respect for
your feelings about the baby.

If you're considering independent adoption, it's

important to have your own lawyer. Adoptive parents
usually will take care of the fees.

Make sure that arrangements are made for counseling. If
you're not getting what you need out of the arrangement,
get another lawyer. With independent adoption, you have
more responsibility to make sure you get the counseling
you need, and that the adoptive parents are pre-screened by
the doctor or lawyer.

In some areas, independent adoption is available through
counseling centers set up for this purpose. It is important
for you to find a service which focuses *first* on the needs of
the birthparents rather than on the adoptive parents.

Rights of Baby's Father

The baby's father must give his permission for adoption.
He could sign a statement denying paternity, sign away his
rights to the child, or give permission for the child to be
adopted. If the father cannot be found, abandonment
proceedings may be carried out.

What if you're making an adoption plan and the birthfather doesn't agree? Counseling may help him understand
why you're making the decision. He may realize he's not
ready to parent a child either.

Ideally, both birthparents agree with the adoption plan.
Maybe the birthfather wants to be with you when you give
birth. Adoption is emotional for everyone involved, and he
may be a source of emotional strength for you. Counseling
can help the birthparents and the adoptive parents work out
their emotions.

What If I Change My Mind?

You can't sign final adoption papers until after your
baby is born. No matter how carefully you decided on
adoption for your child before s/he was born, you will

probably find you need to make your decision all over
again after you deliver. It's best not to make a final decision immediately after you deliver, especially if it's
different from what you had planned.

It's a good idea to write out your reasons for choosing
adoption. Take your list to the hospital so you can look at it
again after you see your baby. If you do decide adoption is
not the right choice for your baby, you certainly can change
your mind. This is true even if you have spent time with the
adoptive parents you chose, and even if they have already
paid some of your bills.

If, when you see your newborn baby, you suddenly feel
the adoption decision is wrong, stall for time. Once again,
go over your reasons for deciding on adoption. Are those
reasons still there? Each state has different adoption laws.
Usually there's a period of time after you have signed the
initial papers when you can change your mind about the
adoption. This is before the adoption is finalized.

Check with a state agency about the laws where you live.
The laws covering agency adoptions may be different than
those concerning independent adoption.

What Will It Cost?

There would be no adoption cost to you except possibly
for medical expenses and your lawyer. The adoptive parents may agree to pay medical expenses and possibly your
living expenses until the baby is born. They also pay any
adoption fees.

Sometimes the adoptive parents offer to give the
birthmother a place to live, either with them or another
family until the baby is born. Adoptive parents can legally
pay for any "reasonable expenses" that you have because of
your pregnancy. They may pay for counseling and your
legal fees.

This may solve a problem for you if you don't have a place to live or money to support yourself until the baby is born. However, an arrangement like this may make you feel pressured if you haven't decided for sure on adoption. You may feel guilty if you change your mind about adoption.

If you do change your mind, you should not have to pay back the money already spent for your medical expenses by the potential adoptive parents.

Pros and Cons

Reasons for adoption:

- Your baby will have a good home and stable family with both a mother and a father.

- You may feel you're not ready to parent a child yet. The adoption option gives you time to mature and grow before starting a family.

- If you do not have resources to care for a baby, or if you currently live in poverty, carrying out an adoption plan may give your baby a better future.

- If you have other problems such as drug abuse, abusive parents or boyfriend, your baby won't have to be involved if s/he's placed for adoption.

Reasons against adoption:

- Adoption is probably the hardest decision to make at the time you're making it. Some young women find that they cannot emotionally let go of their babies and place them with an adoptive family.

- You are aware of what it takes to parent a child, you are realistic about it, and you are prepared to handle these responsibilities.

- You feel that you can give your baby a good home.

- You know that if you made an adoption plan, you would change your mind later.

Questions to Ask Yourself

- Am I emotionally ready to make an adoption decision?

- Are my parents against it? This doesn't mean that adoption is wrong for you, but you need to include your parents in the counseling.

- Are my friends pressuring me to keep the baby?

- Will I go to a reputable agency and assure that the baby is placed in a good home? Or will I work with a reliable independent adoption counseling service?

- Do I have secret plans of going back for the baby later?

- Do I know that I am not ready for the responsibility of caring for and raising a baby?

With counseling, you can resolve all these issues. Adoption is a loving choice. The *right* reason to make an adoption plan is to place the baby in a good home where s/he will be provided with better emotional and physical care than you can provide at this time, and to allow you to continue your life.

Adoption is as much a commitment as keeping and raising a baby. You need to understand that once the adoption is final, you can't get your baby back.

To learn more about adoption including legal aspects, and to read about pregnant women's reasons for making an adoption plan, see *Pregnant? Adoption Is an Option* (1997: Morning Glory Press).

Parents, Pregnant Teens and the Adoption Option: Help for Families (1989: Morning Glory Press) is written for parents of pregnant teens considering the adoption option. You might want to suggest that your parents read it. Doing so could help them deal with their feelings concerning the possible adoption of your baby—and their grandchild.

Adoption Isn't Easy

Sometimes things hurt even when you know it's the right thing to do. Pregnant women bond with their babies before the birth. If you release your baby for adoption you'll feel a sense of loss, and you'll grieve for your baby.

This doesn't mean you made a bad decision. You may find that spending time with your baby before presenting her to the adoptive parents will help.

> *It was definitely a traumatic experience, the hardest thing I ever did. If it hadn't been for Elaine (counselor), I would never have made it. I learned you have to heal. You have to cry, you have to grieve. That's part of the healing process.*
>
> Nancy

Some people plan a presentation ceremony. The birthparents invite close friends and relatives to participate as they formally present their baby to the adoptive parents. They say this helps them accept the fact that someone else is parenting their child.

Most birthparents say that making an adoption plan was the hardest thing they ever had to do. They are comforted in knowing that their baby is having a good life and chances they could not provide. They are able to get on with their lives and continue growing and maturing.

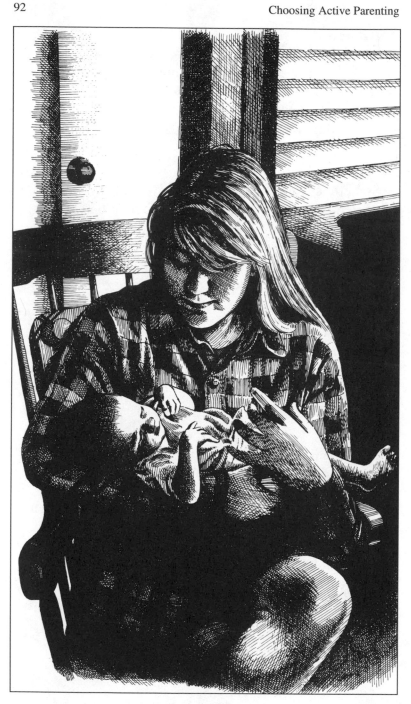

CHAPTER **6**

CHOOSING
ACTIVE PARENTING

There's a lot involved in being a mom. Mostly it takes time—time that you're used to having for yourself. That's my biggest problem with being a mom—no time to myself. I can't even relax and take a bath for five minutes without having to listen to Stephanie crying or worrying about where she is. I can't just sit and read or watch TV because I need to keep an eye on her constantly. Once I finally get her to bed, I have to do my homework and get to bed myself!

It's worth it though, especially when she gives me a hug and a kiss and says, "I love you, Mommy." I can't help but forget all the naughty things she does or how much work she is. That makes me feel so special—and happy, too.

Kate, 17, mother of Stephanie, 14 months

When you decide to keep and raise your baby, you choose instant adulthood. When you become a parent, you choose to leave behind a part of yourself that was more carefree, had few obligations or responsibilities, and had a lot of personal freedom.

When you decide to keep your baby, you make promises to your child and to all others involved that you'll do your best to provide a good home.

You're not giving up your goals and dreams, but you're taking the responsibility for this baby. You know you may have to work harder and with more persistence to realize your dreams and goals. You're agreeing to be a role model, a support system, and protector to another human being.

You're agreeing to accept help from others, such as parents, friends, and outside support groups to help you be a good mother as well as the best person you can become. You're agreeing to design and shape your life as well as helping your child design and shape his or her life.

When you become a parent, you give up some of the freedoms that childhood brings and accept the responsibilities of adulthood. It means sometimes staying home with a sick child instead of going to that party with your friends. It means having to buy diapers and formula instead of CDs and new shoes.

What Are Your Options?

If you want to keep the baby, your options are:

- Raise the baby alone (usually with the help of family or friends).
- You and the father parent together, but not marry now.
- Marry the baby's father and raise the baby together.

We'll talk about these options.

Keeping the Baby and Staying Single

Many teens who keep their babies must do so without
the baby's father. Sometimes the baby's father is no longer
on the scene, or he is not capable of getting married and
supporting a family, or he chooses not to do so.

Most unmarried teenage mothers (and many married
ones) must live with parents or other relatives until they
become self-sufficient. In many cases this means years. I
lived with my parents until I was twenty-one.

During this time, I finished high school, two years of
college, and held several full and part-time jobs. It was
rough going at times for both me and my parents. They
became very attached to my child, and it was traumatic for
everyone (including my daughter) when we moved away.

Despite all this, my parents were supportive and allowed
me to mature (which I desperately needed) and work on my
future. I can't imagine how I would have survived on my
own, although there is public aid available for young
mothers in some states. Public aid, however, never ad-
equately covers housing and other expenses of raising
a child.

I urge you to accept the support of your friends and
family. At the same time, you need to grow toward
becoming self-sufficient and independent.

It usually takes patience on everyone's part. You may
feel you don't have as much freedom and privacy as you'd
like. Your family may feel that they've lost freedom, too.

Parenting

Most single mothers find parenting challenging because
they have a special set of problems and issues to deal with.
Many times girls look forward to parenting the baby because they believe this means they will never be lonely
again. They feel they'll have someone to love who will
return their love.

Sometimes those rewards of being a parent don't come until later, after the baby has received love and care *from* you. Parents have to give a lot of love and care to get anything back. Some teen moms find themselves feeling lonely and isolated because they spend all their time caring for a newborn baby. This feeling usually comes and goes.

Single Parenting Issues

- What about dating? Will I be able to go out with friends or go out on a date?

- How will my boyfriend feel about my baby?

- Will I be able to recognize and protect my child against abuse?

- How will I handle frustration and loneliness that sometimes come with single parenting?

- How do I find out about taking care of a child? There's a lot to know about health, nutrition, discipline, and the emotional care of a child.

- What about money? How much can my parents contribute? How will I pay for child care? Can the baby's father contribute? Or am I pretty much on my own?

If you decide to parent your baby, you'll learn some of these things along the way. If your parents are going to help you, they might be able to give you advice. If you'd like to read about parenting babies and toddlers, including lots of comments from teen parents, see *Teens Parenting,* a helpful four-book series on the topic (1991: Morning Glory Press).

What About the Baby's Father?

Dealing with the baby's father is sometimes complicated. If he's not around, what will you tell the baby about his father? It's best to stay positive because your baby will identify with his father as part of himself.

Do I Have a Daddy? (1991: Morning Glory Press) is a picture book for the child with a missing father. The book includes a section of suggestions for single parents.

Some fathers don't offer marriage or commitment, but instead offer their "presence." Some teen fathers seem supportive and excited during the pregnancy, but lose interest when the baby arrives.

He may feel you spend more time with the baby than with him. This happens to many new fathers. Sometimes with teen fathers it's enough to cause them to quit trying. Maybe you'll continue to date, or he'll drop by on a regular basis to see the baby. This may allow the child to develop a relationship with him.

> *You can't force the father to stay around. After you have the baby, it has a lot to do with you. I've talked with some mothers who don't want the father around. They can't stand him, and they don't want his input.*
>
> *I think the father should have the right to play the dad, to have some say as to what happens to his child. If he isn't going to be around, he should still take some responsibility.*
>
> Cathi, 18, mother of Susie, 18 months

It's also possible that your family does not approve of your relationship with the baby's father. They may be afraid of a repeat pregnancy, or they may feel that the pregnancy was his fault.

This situation can become stressful and complicated for you. You may not know exactly where you stand in your relationship with your baby's father. Maybe he can't help you with money, but could he share his time? Perhaps he could babysit sometimes, or help you with laundry. *Teen Dads: Rights, Responsibilities and Joys* (1993: Morning

Glory Press) is a parenting guide for fathers, whether married, living with the child's mother, or neither.

Fathers play an important role in children's lives. It's wise to put his name on the birth certificate as the father, whether or not you want the baby to use his name.

Establishing paternity early is important both for you and for the baby, and it may help the dad feel more responsibility. It will help your baby with his or her identity. This may also help you get financial support from the father when he becomes able to contribute.

Getting Married

This idea may seem attractive to you. If you're in love with the father, you might jump at marriage if he asks. Marriage, however, is not always the easiest option although he may truly love you and feel a sense of responsibility toward you and the baby.

However, many teenage marriages fail because neither person is ready for the overwhelming responsibility of an early marriage.

This happened to Cara and Tom:

Me and Tom were engaged, and I had told my friends we were getting married in five years. But when I got pregnant, we got married the next week. I think if we had waited, it might have worked. I felt there was something I missed, so I divorced him, and I dated a lot. But that wasn't fun.

We tried to get back together, but by that time, Tom had changed. He was now a single man. He was feeling fine until the divorce, and then he realized he was missing something.

I was never independent. I went straight from an over-protective Mexican father to a husband, so I'm

enjoying this freedom. But if I can find the right
person, I'd prefer marriage.

Cara, now 22, mother of Leroy, 6; Paul, 4; and Nicole, 3

Unless you have parents who provide you both with a
good start, it's a struggle. There may be little joy because
there is neither time nor money to have fun and enjoy each
other. It becomes a struggle for survival.

Often the woman has even more responsibility because
she may feel responsible for the care of the whole household including all cooking, cleaning, shopping, etc. A baby
requires most of her time and attention, and her partner
feels neglected or jealous. (This happens also in marriages
between older couples.)

The woman becomes doubly stressed because she's
trying to raise a baby and hold their relationship together.
Little wonder that many couples break up after living
together for awhile, and that eighty percent of teenage
marriages end in divorce.

Despite all these drawbacks, many young women try
marriage or living together if the opportunity arises. Be
sure to talk about what you each expect from this relationship. Do you want *him* to take care of you and the baby?

Do you think he wants *you* to care for him, feed him, and
cook for him? Some young women say that having a
husband at that age is like having *two* children to care for.
Before you make a final decision, make sure you talk
together about what you both want and expect out of
the marriage or living-together relationship.

Reading *Teenage Couples: Caring, Commitment, and
Change* and *Teenage Couples: Coping with Reality* (1995:
Morning Glory Press) together can help you consider some
of the problems of early marriage and/or moving in together. The books also provide lots of suggestions for making early relationships work in spite of possible obstacles.

Weighing the Good and the Bad

There are good things and bad things about being a parent. Some things are harder when you're young and still not independent. Looking at some of the pros and cons of being a parent at a young age may help:

Pros

- You may feel you can't give up your child. You don't want someone else to raise him or her.

- Parenthood has many rewards although you have to look for the rewards and sometimes wait for them. You'll have to *give* time, love, and care before you get these things back.

- You have an opportunity to "prove" your strength, determination, and persistence.

- You have the opportunity to shape your child's future.

- Although needing to grow up is a poor reason to have a child, the responsibility of children matures and "grounds" you (and I do mean that in both senses of the word).

Cons

- You need a lot of emotional and physical stamina to care for a child for eighteen-plus years. New-borns are particularly demanding, requiring 24-hour-a-day care.

- You will have to make changes in your life. If you were going to go away to college, you may have to live at home and go to a local college. If you were going to move out of your parent's home at 18, you

may have to delay until you're self-sufficient.
You'll have another person to think about.

- You give up being a teenager to become an adult.
  This means dealing with adult problems and
  bypassing some of the joys of being a teenager.

- You give up a good deal of your usual freedom.
  You become responsible for another human being.
  You won't be able to go out as much with friends.
  You won't be able to spend all your money on
  yourself.

- You may delay your independence. It takes more
  resources and energy to become independent if you
  are already a parent. It may be tougher to finish
  school.

- More than half of all women on welfare were
  teenage mothers. You have to be determined and
  ambitious to break away from the poverty cycle.

- Your child could become a target for child abuse.
  Young mothers have to deal with the frustrations of
  parenting. Also, boyfriends may not know how to
  deal with a child.
  When you become a parent, you make a promise
  to protect your baby's safety. It means saying
  goodbye to an abusive boyfriend, or asking for help
  from a counselor if you feel you're not coping.

- You'll have to look harder and longer for a new
  relationship that suits you *and* your baby. It takes
  an exceptional man to shoulder the extra responsibility and to love your child. You'll have to be
  more selective. Your baby's well-being and safety
  become your primary concern, and your needs
  become secondary.

Questions to Ask Yourself

- Do I have family and friends who are willing to help?

- Do I want to keep the baby only because my boyfriend (or someone else) wants me to?

- Do I have the emotional and physical stamina to care for a baby 24 hours a day?

- Do I have the courage and determination to pursue my goals and still raise my child, perhaps without a father?

- What if my baby has special needs? Mental retardation, birth defects, epilepsy, and birth injuries occur more often among children born to teenage mothers. While odds are that I will have a healthy baby, "What would I do if . . . ?"

- If I'm getting married, is he mature enough to stick with us?

- Has my boyfriend ever threatened or hurt me in any way?

- Do I keep thinking I can change my mind if I don't really want to be a mom?

- Do I have thoughts that what I really want to do is go out at night and have fun like the rest of the kids?

- Do I have fantasies that my mother or someone else will take care of the baby for me?

- Do I believe that my boyfriend will come back if I keep this baby?

- If you are very young (under sixteen), it will be
  even harder for you. You're further away from
  independence than older pregnant teens. You
  probably don't have as many skills as the older girl
  for coping with problems of a baby, and you'll have
  to depend on your parents and others even more.

Why Is the "Con" List Longer?

Deciding to parent a baby is a big commitment. Most
parents, married or not, could make a list of reasons not to
have children. Maybe their list would be longer than the
reasons to have children. But the rewards are there, and
that's why couples continue to have children.

My life is different than a year ago, but I like it bet-
ter now. I didn't go out much before I got pregnant. I
think some teenage parents are miserable because
they make it miserable. They don't try hard enough.

To become a parent, to raise a child, is not easy.
But if you try, while you can't make it easy, you can
make it fun. I have a lot of fun with him. It's only
miserable if you make it miserable.

Liz, 16, mother of Jonathan, three months

It's good to think about all the aspects of parenting a
child. All these things will help you decide if you're ready
to handle the challenges of parenting.

Ask yourself the questions in the box on the opposite
page. These, without a doubt, are some of the most important questions you will consider in your entire life. Answering them carefully and honestly will help you get on with
your decision-making.

Now that you know about your options and you know
some questions to ask yourself, the next chapter will help
you understand how to make these important decisions.

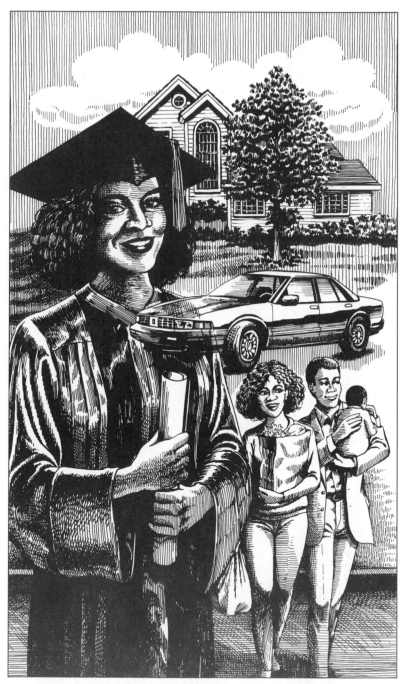

CHAPTER 7

IT'S *YOUR* DECISION

Dear Shirley,
   I'm sixteen and seven months pregnant. At first, my parents wanted me to have an abortion, but I didn't want one. My boyfriend wants me to raise the baby with his help.
   *I'm not sure what **I** want. My feelings seem to change from day to day. Should I make my boyfriend happy? No wonder I'm confused.*

April

Anyone would be confused in this situation. April must make her own decision, but that doesn't mean she can't listen to advice from others.

Maybe knowing *how* to make a decision would make it easier for April—and for you.

How Do You Decide?

You may have made a lot of decisions already. In some families, the children have responsibilities at a young age. Maybe your family let you pretty much run your own life. If that's the case, you've had experience making decisions. All you need is to know more about your choices.

If you're used to having others make decisions for you, you'll need to know *how* to make a decision first.

When you can answer the following questions, you've followed the steps to making a decision:

1) What are my choices?

2) What information do I need about each choice?

3) What are the good things about each choice?

4) What are the bad things about each choice?

5) Weigh the good things and the bad things.

6) Make a decision.

7) How do I feel about the decision?

You can repeat the steps as many times as you need to. You can change your mind as long as the options are still available to you.

Don't Give Your Decision Power Away

Sometimes when you need to make a decision, it seems easier to let someone else take control. You may give away your decision power without realizing it. This may happen if you:

• **Don't make a decision.**
  You're letting too much time pass. You're not doing anything to decide, and finally you accept your fate. What will happen if April doesn't decide?

- **Let someone else decide.**
  It may seem easier to let your mother or boyfriend
  decide for you. You love them, so you want to
  please them. Or, maybe a friend seems to know a
  lot about your problem, and you want her to decide.

- **Make the most popular decision.**
  Some people believe there is one *right* thing to do.
  Maybe in your family, anyone who gets pregnant
  has the baby and parents. Maybe where you live, a
  pregnant teen is expected to parent her baby. Does
  that make it harder to decide on adoption?

It's *Your* Decision

What if you let your parents decide? Maybe your emotions tell you that's not the right thing to do, and you feel
bad about the decision. You left one important person out
of the decision—*you*. Here's what one young woman
thinks about making your own decisions:

> *Hold your head up high. If somebody doesn't like
> it, too bad. You can't let what people say and think
> get you down because then you would be down all the
> time. You really have to grow and be a strong person.*
> Margie, 19, mother of Art, 3

Repeat pregnancies sometimes happen to girls who
regret the decision they made. They have a desire to "do it
right next time." It's much better to resolve your feelings
with this pregnancy than to go through the whole thing
again.

Others Are Affected

Sometimes you may *want* to be alone. You'd like other
people to leave you alone, but they don't. Suddenly, you're
the topic of conversation around the dinner table at night.

Or, you overhear your mom talking on the phone with a friend about what you should or should not do.

If you think about it, though, whatever you decide could change the lives of several people.

Your Baby

If you decide to have your baby, you'll choose between parenting your baby or making an adoption plan. Babies are very needy. They need someone to care constantly for them, both physically and emotionally. Caring for a baby takes time and money.

If you decide to parent the baby yourself, you'll need your family or friends to support you financially and emotionally. Some girls decide to make an adoption plan because they realize they cannot give their baby all the things a baby needs.

As a parent, you know your baby's needs come before your own. The baby will depend on you for safety, comfort, and health. If you are dating someone you like very much, but who threatens your baby in any way, you have to choose not to see him. If your baby needs new shoes and you want a pair of jeans, you may have to wait for the jeans. Your baby deserves to be loved, to be protected, and to be given the best chance possible.

Your Parents and Family

My parents argue every night about what we should do. It's almost like I don't have a say. It's depressing. I keep changing my mind about what to do.
                                        Jodi, pregnant at 16

Your parents are probably upset and confused. They might be so upset that they want to make the decision themselves. If you have a strong feeling about what you want to do, talk to them about it. Sometimes parents react with comments such as these:

- "Where did I fail?"
- "How could you do this to us?"
- "You'll have to have it and keep it. You asked for it, now you have it."
- "You must get an abortion immediately. There's no way you can raise a baby."
- "Friends and relatives mustn't find out about this. Abortion is the only solution."
- "You'll have to have the baby and give it up. We don't believe in abortion."

Most parents cry, get depressed, or get excited, sometimes to the point of violence. This stage usually doesn't last very long. They'll adjust just like you will. Your parents have reason to be concerned about your decision because they will be affected, especially if you decide to keep the child.

Most young women need help with money and emotional support. Most pregnant teenagers who do not marry will live with parents or other relatives, sometimes for years. Some who marry will still have to live with parents because of limited money.

Some of the ways your parents will most likely have to help if you keep your baby:

- Additional room for the baby.
- Money for baby food, formula, diapers, clothes, and other baby items if you can't provide them.
- Medical care for you and the baby—often not covered by insurance.
- Babysitting or daycare expenses while you go to school or work.

- Additional emotional support for you and for baby.

- They'll have to change their lifestyle. There will be baby toys on the floor and a noisier household. They may find themselves taking care of the baby instead of going on that trip they've planned.

You may want to suggest they read *School-Age Parents: The Challenge of Three-Generation Living* (1990: Morning Glory Press). It's written especially for parents whose teenage daughter brings her baby home to live.

In addition to offering this book to your parents, you might like to read it. You might gain some insight into the way your parents may feel about your pregnancy and about having your child living with them.

How do *you* feel about being dependent on your parents for a period of time? Discuss your feelings in detail with them. Don't be afraid of hurting them further because it would be even worse to do something you don't want.

Your brothers and sisters are also affected by your decision. They may be afraid for you, or embarrassed. They may even be jealous of the extra attention you're getting. Will they talk to you about their feelings?

Your Friends

Your friends are affected by your pregnancy because they may not be able to see you as much. You may not be able to do some of the things you did before you became pregnant.

Even my parents say they're going to take Myles away from me because I like to go out. But that's natural, I'm young. But they think I should stay home all the time. It's hard to get friends with a baby, and it's hard to get a boyfriend. Sometimes I feel like

*sitting down and crying. I meet a guy, tell him I have
a kid, and he says goodbye.*

Janette, 18, mother of Myles, 7 months

Friends may offer to babysit. They say they'll come and
change diapers for you, but they may not help as often as
you'd like. Your friends have their own lives. They may
seem excited about the baby during your pregnancy and
when they see your newborn, but then may back away.

Some things about having a baby are not fun. They keep
you from seeing your friends as much as before. They keep
you at home.

Not all your friends will desert you, and you'll probably
find new friends, too. Your friends are an important source
of emotional support, and you can bounce some of your
feelings off them. Try to figure out what your friend's
motives are when they push you for a certain decision.
Some examples:

- Susie wants you to have an abortion because *she*
  had one and she believes it's the best thing to do.

- Jane wants you to keep the baby because they're so
  cute and she wants to know someone who has one.

- Mary thinks you should give the baby up for
  adoption because she's adopted and look how well
  she turned out!

- Maria says it would be terrible for you to have an
  abortion because she doesn't believe in abortion.

- Janice wants you to get married because she thinks
  that would be *so* romantic.

These are all reasons why *your friend* would benefit
from the decision either by providing something she wants,
or by making *her* decision seem right.

Sometimes, of course, friends give *good* advice. We need friends to share thoughts and ideas, but *not* to make our decisions for us.

Your Boyfriend

If your boyfriend is still in the picture, it's usually up to you how involved you want him to be. You need his permission to carry out an adoption plan.

What if he tells you that if you have the baby, he will help you parent? Even if he tells you now that he'll be around to help you raise the baby, he may change his mind later.

> *My boyfriend, he's not really saying what he wants.*
> *He comes around and we talk, but we don't go out*
> *like we used to. I don't know what he's thinking very*
> *much. Sometimes he seems proud, but other times, I*
> *just think he's mad or something.*

Lara, pregnant at 17

Your baby's father is probably confused too. He may be torn by feelings of love and responsibility for you and feelings of fear.

If he's willing, talking to a counselor together might help the two of you sort out your feelings. Fathers play an important role in parenting. If he's willing to work at it, your child could benefit.

Listen To Your Fantasies

What do you picture when you fantasize about you and the baby? Some fantasies indicate that you are not ready to accept the responsibility of caring for a baby:

*   The baby's father will come back and we'll probably get married.

- My mom or my sister will love the baby so much that they'll want to take care of him all the time. Then I can still go out the way I do now.

- I'll have the baby and keep him for a while. If it gets too much for me to handle, someone will take him off my hands.

- I've always loved dolls. It will be fun having a baby to dress up and take places.

Having these fantasies does not mean that you would be a lousy mother or that you're a terrible person. They only mean that you might need to think more clearly about your options.

What will happen if your fantasy comes true? What if it doesn't? These kinds of thoughts indicate that you realize the extent of the job of caring for a baby:

- I'll be able to go out some, but not nearly as much as now.

- My friends may not stay around to help me. If they don't, I'll still be okay.

- Chances are, I'll never see my boyfriend again, but I'll still love and care for my baby.

- I know it won't be easy taking care of a baby. S/he'll have a lot of needs. I'll need help for awhile.

Every woman has fantasies about her baby before it's born, about what it looks like and how it will behave. These kinds of thoughts are normal. Your fantasies can tell you how you really feel and what you want for your future.

Role-Play Your Choices

You may have tried role-playing at school or in some other group. When you role-play, you pretend you are already in a certain situation.

> *We did this thing when I was in Junior High where we had to take an egg with us everywhere we went like it was a baby. We colored little faces on it and everything. Sometimes being a mother is like that, you have to always remember it and take care of it.*
>
> Jeri, age 18, mother of Gina, age 2

You could offer to babysit for a friend or relative. If possible, keep the baby for the weekend or longer. That'll give you time to see what it's like to care for a baby. How do you feel?

How would you feel if you couldn't give the baby back to its mother? Was caring for the baby about what you expected? Role-play helps you understand how you'll feel after your decision.

What Would You Do If?

Sometimes pretending "what if" helps you know if you're making this decision by yourself, or if someone else is influencing you too much. This exercise is good for people-pleasers. If you're a people-pleaser, you may spend a lot of time trying to figure out what would make other people happy.

You may think, "What does mom want me to do?" Or, "What does Jeff really want?" Blanking them out for a while may help you decide on the best alternative for you and your baby:

- What would you do if your boyfriend disappeared? Would your decision be the same?

- What if your parents weren't in the picture? Pretend that you don't have parents, or that they don't care what you do.

Put Yourself in the Future

Try to picture yourself five years in the future. Is there a child there? Remember that s/he would not be a baby, s/he would be a small person.

If you're sixteen now, ten years from now you'll be twenty-six and your baby will be ten. How do you feel about having a ten-year-old? What are you doing? How do you feel about your child? Are your friends in the picture? What about your boyfriend? Are you married? Do you have other children?

If It Hurts, Is It Wrong?

No. Most young mothers grieve no matter what they decide. If you decide on adoption or abortion, you may grieve for your baby. If you decide to parent your child, you will grieve for the life you used to have.

No matter what you decide, you may long for the time when your life wasn't so complicated. Grief hurts. The hurt will be less as time goes on, and you'll find ways to turn the pain into good things.

What If You Decide Wrong?

You *cannot* decide wrong. There are no easy answers, but there is more than one right response. You might change your mind many times during your pregnancy, but you *will* make a decision, accept it, and get on with life.

Give yourself a pat on the back for making that decision *on your own*.

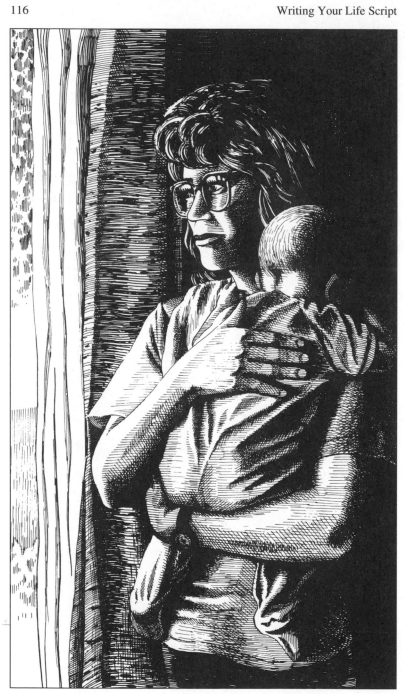

Introduction

PART THREE

WRITING YOUR LIFE SCRIPT

A few years ago, a respected social scientist made this statement:

> *"The girl who has an illegitimate child at the age of 16 suddenly has 90 percent of her life's script written for her. She will probably drop out of school; even if someone in her family helps to take care of the baby, she will probably not be able to find a steady job that pays enough to provide for herself and her child; she may feel impelled to marry someone she might not otherwise have chosen. Her life choices are few, and most of them are bad."* (1987: *Adolescent Mothers in Later Life*, Cambridge University Press).

How does this passage make you feel? Does it make you feel hopeful? Probably not. Let's rewrite this script:

As a pregnant teenager, being young, resourceful, and resilient, you can write your own life script. You can stay in school, go to college, and find many things rewarding and educational about your situation. You can look at this as a challenge to be used as a tool for emotional, personal, and spiritual growth. You can marry the person who is right for you, or not marry at all if that's what you wish. Although your chosen path may vary from the one you originally planned, your choices are many, your opportunity for growth great.

Although you may not have planned on this pregnancy, many good things will come out of your experience. You'll learn and grow. Others around you will learn and grow. The next chapters suggest things you can do to write your own life script.

CHAPTER 8

SOCIAL INSECURITY— BOYFRIENDS, OTHERS

"Nobody can make you feel inferior without your consent." —Eleanor Roosevelt

Jennifer

Jennifer was sixteen when she had her baby. She was devastated when she learned she was pregnant. Her boyfriend left, and she grieved for the relation-ship for a while. She decided to keep the baby because her mother was willing to help her finish high school and go on to college. Jennifer hoped her boyfriend would return and they would become a family.

Two months before her baby was born, Jennifer became excited about the baby, which she was sure was a boy. Secretly, she thought that having a boy would make her boyfriend come back. She began

preparing for the baby, buying baby clothes with her mother and preparing the room that she and the baby would share. Jennifer's friends seemed excited about her pregnancy and the baby.

Jennifer had a little girl who was small and wrinkled and cried all the time. Jennifer fell into a deep depression, but was unable to talk to anyone about it. After all, they'd think she was a monster for wanting a little boy and for not thinking her baby was pretty. Jennifer is overwhelmed and resentful of her situation. Sometimes she fantasizes that the baby gets sick and dies. That makes Jennifer even more depressed.

Jennifer's mother sometimes acts embarrassed about the baby, even though she loves her grand-daughter. Once, Jennifer heard her tell a stranger in the grocery store that the baby was hers.

Jennifer's friends stopped coming around often. When they did, they acted distant and hurried. She misses being able to go out with them and just have fun without worrying about the baby at home. Even though Jennifer has her family and her baby, she is lonely.

What Should Jennifer Do?

Much of what Jennifer feels has to do with how others react to her situation. Strangers and new friends are curious. Some young men are reluctant to date someone with a small child. Old friends have drifted away.

It may take Jennifer some time to work out her problems and build a future for herself and her child. She needs to avoid doing anything out of desperation. She has time on her side, and she can use it to her advantage. Time will allow her to learn and grow.

With time, Jennifer will learn that some people will
admire her for what she's doing, and some people will not.
Some young men will be patient and loving with her
daughter, and others will not. Jennifer will learn to recognize someone who is not good for her and her baby. When
this happens, she'll say goodbye to that person.

To get moving on a positive forward track, Jennifer
should talk to someone about what she's feeling. She could
share her feelings with a teen mom group or a trusted
friend. Even more important, she should keep trying, keep
asking for help until she gets some direction.

Your Friends

*I can't do what I used to do. I can't just go out and
do stuff with my friends like I used to. There's a few
friends that stuck around, that'll come over sometimes. Then there's my new friends. You have to find
new friends. I don't want to party all the time now.*

Sharon, 17, mother of Leif, 13 months

If your friends have drifted away, it's probably not that
they're deserting you. Instead, you may be drifting away
from each other. Your life is changing, so you have a new
need for supportive friends.

Perhaps your friend's parents won't allow you at their
house anymore. They may act as though your pregnancy is
contagious. They're probably afraid it might happen to
their daughter, too.

You may long for your old relationship with your family. Even if they're supportive and helpful, it's not the same
as it was when you were younger and didn't have a child of
your own.

*Connie's friends were a comfort to her during her
pregnancy. They went shopping with her for maternity*

*clothes, helped her pick out names for the baby, and
one friend even volunteered to be her labor coach.*

*After the baby was born, however, her friends
drifted away. They came to see the baby a few times,
but they quit asking Connie to go out because she was
"always busy with the baby." They still called sometimes, but Connie said, "I felt like they were forcing
themselves to talk to me."*

Connie is discovering that relationships change and
evolve depending on what happens in our lives. Friendships
may change because of different needs and wants. You may
have evolved to a different level of maturity and responsibility than your friends. Maybe it scares them a little?

It's possible that you don't have much money and time
to go to movies and to party. Maybe you don't fit in with
the old group anymore. Sometimes their parents discourage
them from seeing you.

For whatever reason, you may sense your old friends are
not right for you anymore. Or, maybe the reverse is true,
and *they* feel that the friendship isn't right.

It's best to see this as *change* and not rejection. If you're
disturbed by the cooling of friendships, talk honestly to
them about it.

Remember how many millions of people there are in the
world. Some of them are going to like you and some of
them won't. Some of your old friends will stand by you,
and some may not.

Think about the possibility of *new* friends. You can
continue to make friends all your life. One of the best ways
to do this is to go to a support group for young women who
have been through what you've been through. Also, remember that you don't have to "stick to your own" and just
associate with other teen mothers. You can meet and make
friends with all kinds of people.

Your Boyfriend

*Guys can just walk away whenever they want to.
Girls can't.*

Cindy, pregnant at 17

*I spend a lot of time trying to figure out what he
wants, whether he's going to come walking back into
my life or not.*

Terry, pregnant at 16

Your boyfriend may no longer be in your life. Or maybe
you're living together, but you don't know where you stand
with him. What if he hangs around, not really in, but not
really out of your life? I was surprised to learn that this
is common.

He may be able to contribute to your life and your
child's life, both emotionally and financially. Just knowing
that he cares could add some emotional stability to your
child's life.

It comes down to asking yourself, "Am I better off with
him or without him?" That's not an easy question to answer. Sometimes our hearts tell us that we need someone,
even when that person is hurting us more than helping.

*I just wish I was older and was married, or even
living with the father. . . I wish he was a father who
wanted to settle down. I pray he will soon. I know he
loves me. He just needs space.*

Frederica, 16, mother of Elias, 5 months

Sometimes a young man becomes confused over pregnancy and fatherhood. Your baby's father may love you,
but be frightened by his responsibility to you. Maybe he
feels he's not ready for marriage.

Some young men talk about wanting to be "friends,"
which is normal in a relationship where you have built

a bond between you. But, if you want something more than a friendship, being told you are a "friend" can be torture to the soul.

Does being your "friend" mean that you cannot date other guys, or that he exerts a certain control over you or your activities? If he acts as a sort of "watchdog," you may find it comforting to think that he cares enough about you to go to all that effort.

How do you know if you should try to make the relationship work? Try weighing the pros and cons. Does the relationship cause you more pain than pleasure?

These things mean the relationship needs work:

- He's nice sometimes, and distant, rude, or even mean or cruel to you at other times.

- You suspect that he's dating other girls.

- He uses noncommittal language like, "I don't know what I want."

- You don't feel good about yourself when you're together.

- You feel he is using you sexually; you don't feel loved or cared about.

- You feel panicky and anxious about the relationship when you're apart. You no longer describe yourself as "happy."

- He is abusive to you or your child.

- He wants to control you, but not take responsibility for you and your child.

- He's not adding to your child's life either by parenting, providing support, or showing interest.

- You feel out of control in the relationship.

If he cares about you, why does he do cruel things to hurt you? He probably truly is confused and is making attempts to push you away, to make you hate him so badly that you end the relationship. If he cannot face up to and talk to you about his feelings, the relationship has little or no chance of surviving.

Frederica, who is quoted earlier, made this statement a couple of months later:

> *I've decided I'm not gonna always be wishing he was here. I have a baby. My boyfriend is a dog, but so what? I love my son, and I'm going to do my best to get my education and be the best mom I can be with or without Elias' father. I don't need him.*

Sometimes relationships become violent because the young woman may want the relationship so much that she becomes submissive. The more submissive she gets, the more her boyfriend abuses her. The more abuse she takes, the weaker her self-image becomes. This is a vicious cycle, and both parties involved need help.

If this is happening to you, reading *Breaking Free From Partner Abuse* by Mary Marecek (1993: Morning Glory Press) might help. Written by the director of a shelter outside of Boston, the underlying message of this 96-page book is "You don't deserve this." *And you don't.*

What If You Decide to Say Goodbye?

Maybe you've weighed the pros and the cons, and you realize that the relationship causes you a lot of pain. So, what do you do? Do you tell him to get lost for good? Do you try to change? It's a question that no one can answer but you.

It's good to give a relationship a chance if the good things about it outweigh the bad. Maybe a friend, relative, or counselor can help you sort out your feelings. Try making a list of the positive things about your relationship. Then, make a list of the negative things. Does one list have more items on it than the other? Does one have *more important* items on it than the other?

Learning to say goodbye to people who no longer give you the love and support you need is not easy. Believe me, it's not easy for adults either. Every person has to say goodbye at some time to someone in her/his life. Simply put, saying goodbye hurts.

So, what can you do? You could get involved in something that interests you. Sometimes when we suffer a loss, we cannot stop thinking about the loss.

Try *not* to think of the color blue. Does this make you keep seeing the color blue in your mind? That's similar to what happens when we lose someone we're close to. That's why keeping busy helps to keep one's mind focused on something else.

Inquiring Minds Want to Know

> *You go to the grocery store and they sort of stare at you. It's not everybody, but they stare at you. Parents mostly.*
>
> *One guy talked about his daughter and asked if I thought it would happen to her. I asked him if she was dating someone. When he said yes, I told him that she was probably having sex. He looked real scared, but I thought he deserved it for asking me.*
>
> Donna, pregnant at 17

People are interested in your situation—what happened, why it happened, who it happened with, and where it happened. They might have young daughters or sons themselves, or possibly they were in a similar situation.

Sometimes it's not a word or a question, it's a look. This attention bothers some girls, and others are not bothered at all. Some young women even like the attention a little.

Your parents may struggle with this, too. They may be worried about how to tell others about your pregnancy. They may try to keep it a secret at first. This is new for them, and they are adjusting, too. Actually, they may find their friends to be more supportive than they expected.

When Smart People Ask Stupid Questions

"It is not every question that deserves an answer."
—Horace

As a teen parent, I've been asked a lot of questions over the years, and I've heard most of them more than once. I used to answer automatically, and I even rehearsed my answers.

The questions haven't changed much.

"How did it happen?"

"How old were you?"

"Did you know who the father was?"

"Were your parents mad?"

"Aren't you afraid you'll be a grandmother before you're forty?"

"How could you *possibly* be her mother?"

"How old are you, and how old is she?" (This last question is followed by a pause while they figure out how old you were when you had the baby.)

Before answering questions, look at the person's reason for asking the question. If they have a daughter, sister, or friend they want to help, you may feel like talking. If you sense that they are going to run to their best friend and retell the story (in their own words), you don't have to talk.

You don't *owe* anyone an explanation. It is your right to

tell as much or as little about yourself as you want to. If someone is trying to help you, such as a counselor, psychologist, or teacher, you should tell them as much as you can about your situation.

Remember, though, that doctors, counselors, psychologists, and teachers are *people,* and they come in many varieties. If you're not comfortable with one or don't like how s/he makes you feel, find another one. Follow your instincts; if the conversation is flowing easily and effortlessly, you are probably talking to the right person.

I have found that if I choose to answer a particular question, if I answer it straightforwardly and honestly, people respect the rest of my privacy and don't press. But, it is *your* choice and *your* right to talk as little or as much as you want about you and your situation.

Before you disclose information about yourself, ask yourself these questions:

- Does talking to this person make me feel better, or worse?

- Do I trust this person? Has he or she betrayed me before?

- Do I sound whiny or dependent when I talk to this person?

- Is this person trying to help me in some way?

- Has the person explained his or her interest in my situation?

Just because someone is older, more educated, or more sophisticated doesn't mean s/he has your best interest in mind. Maybe he's biased against adoption, abortion, or a teenager with a baby. Maybe she's personally angry at someone in her past. Maybe he's just curious. You don't want to be distrustful, but you don't want to give away your self-respect either.

If you don't want to answer, or if the question makes you feel bad, just walk away. A simple "I'm sorry, but I just don't feel like talking about it," will solve the problem. Or you could say, "It's a long story and I don't have time to get into it."

Talking Can Help

There are some wonderful groups for pregnant teenagers or teens who have dropped out of school and want to return. Check with your local high school or social services.

If you consider yourself an organizer, why not start your own group? Other teens will appreciate it, and you'll get a chance to exercise your leadership talents.

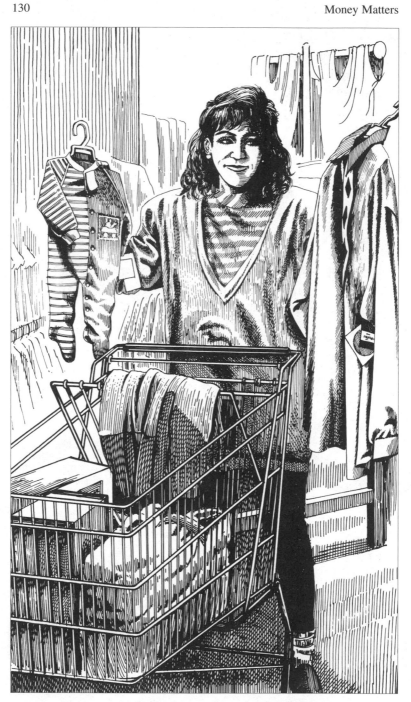

CHAPTER 9

MONEY MATTERS

"It seems my biggest problem is money. I can buy food and diapers, but that's it."

Sharon, 17, mother of Leif, 13 months

"Prices have gone up terribly. Clothing is very expensive. It's hard because I'm unemployed. Little shoes cost so much, almost as much as mine. I've been trying to save and get enough money for an apartment, but then rents go up again.

Dolores, 19, mother of Jeremiah, 3

Does money matter? Money really doesn't buy happiness, but the lack of "enough" money can cause a lot of unhappiness. As you know, everyone needs a certain amount of money for food, a place to live, clothes to wear, and a little fun.

Think about some of the famous single moms, like Cher and Goldie Hawn. Do they worry about how to buy groceries or how to pay the rent next month? Probably not. Not having to worry about money allows them freedom to think about other things for their children. Having money also changes the opinions that others have toward them.

It's not really the *money* that matters, but the freedom and opportunity it provides. It's good to think about how you'll make money, and how you'll spend it. Most young women dream of an apartment of their own, but it doesn't come easy:

> *I don't want to stay here because I don't get along very well with my parents. But to get an apartment costs $1000 to move in the door. I can't possibly do it on welfare.*
>
> *Most places I call tell me they won't even accept children. I don't know what I'm going to do. Maybe I can find a roommate, but that's hard when you have a child. I wish I could have waited about six more years. Myles isn't a toy.*
>
> Janette, 18, mother of Myles, 7 months

You may not have thought much about the money situation because you're still living with your parents, family, or friends. Your parents or family, however, may feel the pressure if you're going to live with them.

Money is sometimes the last thing you think of when you're upset about being pregnant. It might help to start thinking and planning what you'll do about money. If you're getting married or moving in together, you and your partner will need to make financial plans together.

Handling Baby Costs

Raising a baby means medical costs, clothing, food, entertainment, toys, education, equipment, and babysitting.

As children grow, their needs change, and your expenses change and increase along with those needs.

It might help to spend some time making a list of things you'll need for the baby. Maybe a friend or your mom can help. Then, price the items. How can you get the cost down? Here are some ideas:

- **Garage sales.** Sometimes you can find like-new baby clothes and things like high chairs, car seats, playpens, and dressing tables.

- **Hand-me-downs.** Do you know someone who has baby items they no longer need? Sometimes friends and family are happy to hand them down.

- **Used items in the paper.** Sometimes you can find bargains by looking in local papers or bulletin boards.

- **Swap with other teen moms.** If you belong to a teen mom group, you could start a pool of used items or exchange items.

- **Buy an item a week.** Sometimes it helps to spread out the expense by picking up a few things each time you're at the store. You could watch for sale items and special deals. Or, if your boyfriend wants to help, ask him to pick up a few things for you whenever he goes to the store.

- **Plan to cut costs.** How can you save money on baby items? Maybe by using cloth diapers instead of expensive disposables. You could breastfeed your baby instead of buying formula.

- **Help from baby's father.** If your boyfriend cannot provide support on a regular basis, is he or his family willing to provide some things for the baby?

Occasional baby food, money for babysitters, baby
clothes, and diapers would help. Let them know
you'd appreciate it. They may be glad to help.

If You're Living with Parents

My parents were upset because they had all these
things they wanted to do. You know, like travel. Now
they say they can't because of me having this baby.

Donna, pregnant at 17

Your parents may be worried about supporting another
child. They may even resent your pregnancy because of the
added expense. Maybe they had planned on retiring soon.
Possibly you live in a one-parent home where money is
already tight.

If both your parents work, they may worry about who
will babysit. If you don't have health insurance to cover
your pregnancy, there will be doctor and hospital bills.

It'll help your family to know that you're thinking about
money matters and planning how to cut costs and help out.
It helps to sit down with them and talk about where the
money will come from, how much they'll contribute, and
what you'll pay for.

If You're Getting Married

Wayne made good money, but we still had money
problems. He was in control of the money and I had
no say-so over it. He said he was doing the work so he
would manage the money—-as if taking care of the
baby wasn't work. I had to ask him if I wanted to
write a check.

Stevie, 18, mother of Leah, 10 months

Getting married doesn't solve money problems. Sometimes it's even harder being married because you and your

partner may have all the responsibility for coming up with money. Money pressures can cause problems between partners.

It's good to talk about earning, budgeting, and spending even before you get married or move in together. Some young women are afraid to "rock the boat" and get him worried about money before the marriage. It's wise, though, to get everything out in the open.

How does he feel about you working? About you going back to school? Is he going to work? How much money will you need? Will you live with parents or friends?

Why finish high school if you're getting married? Today it usually takes two incomes to support a family. You probably will need to work to contribute to family income, or you may need to provide the main family income. What if your husband loses his job? What if you get a divorce? What if you simply *want* to work away from home?

Finishing high school will give your self-esteem a boost as well as provide a good example for your child. It will help you feel less dependent on your husband and others.

Childcare

Childcare may be your biggest expense. Even if you're living with your parents, they may not be home during the day to babysit while you work or go to school. You may find you need to go to school during the day and work in the evening, or vice versa. Maybe your family doesn't feel physically or emotionally capable of babysitting for extended periods. This means many hours that your child will need out-of-family care.

Some young moms are lucky to have relatives who are willing to babysit for them, at least for part of the day. Does your school have a teen mom program that provides day care for infants? Does your church provide babysitting?

Can you trade babysitting with other teen moms? Is there a way you can work at home to earn money? Do you qualify for public aid to assist with daycare expenses?

You may get frustrated trying to find good care for your child. Don't give up though; your education is worth it.

Learning to Budget

I'm a pretty good money manager because I have to be. When I get my check, I pay my bills first, then I buy groceries, usually $50 a week. I buy meat first, then vegetables, then canned food. I usually use fresh vegetables because they're a lot cheaper. The only thing I buy that's junk is popsicles.

Roseanna, 15, mother of Felipe, 2

Budgeting is usually a matter of stretching your money to meet your expenses. Decisions must be made. Essential things, like food and childcare, must be paid first. Then, if there's money left, it can go for entertainment and clothes.

Most young people want to be independent and to live on their own as soon as possible. To get an idea of the costs of running a household, check local prices for rent, utilities, daycare, and car expenses.

Ask your parents how much their basic bills are every month. This can give you an idea of how much it would cost you to live on your own. From this, you'll know how much you need to make to support yourself.

If you have some money, it's wise to get a checking account and learn to balance it every month. Credit cards are good for establishing credit and for emergencies, but you won't want to use them to live on. Many people get into trouble using credit cards like money. When you use one, you're spending your future earnings.

It's helpful to draw up a simple budget. Maybe you're

working and living at home and your parents will provide some support. You'll still need to decide where your money will go. Even if your parents pay for part of your food and they don't charge you rent, you'll have expenses.

Here's a sample monthly budget:

INCOME	EXPENSES
$300.00	$75.00(food)
(part-time job)	25.00(clothes)
	125.00 (childcare)
	50.00 (medical for baby)
	25.00 (entertainment)
TOTAL $300.00	$300.00

Budgeting is simply making income equal expenses. You only have so much to spend, and that's it. Some months you have "surprise" bills. Maybe your car needs new tires, or your child is sick a lot that month and you have more medical bills. Sometimes credit cards help with these surprise bills, but they shouldn't be used for things for which you could wait.

Public Aid

If you're on your own, or your family is low-income, you may qualify for AFDC—Aid to Families with Dependent Children. It may be a short-term solution to serious money problems.

Check with your local Social Services Department. In some states it's hard for minors to get welfare when they have parents who are responsible for them. Although welfare is a good temporary relief from poverty, it's not a long-term solution:

Sometimes I run out of money. There is no way I
can rely on welfare. My cousin said, "I'm going to
get pregnant and get on welfare." I told her she
was crazy.

Leslie, 20, mother of Kenny, 4 months, and Amy, 2

Your local health department can tell you if you're
eligible for WIC (Women, Infant and Children food program). WIC provides coupons for milk and other nutritious
foods for pregnant women and babies.

Is there subsidized housing in your area? Section 8, a
federally funded program through HUD (Housing and
Urban Development), allows the Housing Aurthority to pay
for part of the rent for the tenant. Call the Housing Department at your city hall and ask if they administer the Section
8 applications.

If you want to attend college after high school, check
on grants and scholarships for women returning to school.
Your local college financial aid department may be able
to help you.

Child Support?

You're probably entitled to child support. Most young
moms don't pursue it for a number of reasons. If your
boyfriend is around your age, he may be in high school
himself. Maybe he doesn't work. It's tough to get money
from someone who doesn't have much.

Maybe you feel responsible for the pregnancy and don't
want to make him pay. Maybe you don't want to make him
mad at you. His family may volunteer assistance with
medical bills or care of the baby. How does *your* family
feel about this? They may be able to assist in smaller ways,
like providing occasional clothing or diapers for the baby.

If you're confused about what the father's responsibilities are, you and your family may want to talk to a lawyer.

If the father is an adult, he definitely should be helping with
financial support now. If he's young and still in school,
maybe he can't help you immediately, but what about a few
years from now?

Your child's needs are important. Deciding not to pursue
child support because of your own feelings could cheat
your child in the future.

Can You Afford School?

It's tough to go to school when you have heavy responsibilities at home. Sometimes school seems like a waste of
time and money. It seems really tough at times to keep
going. Try to take one day at a time and stick with it. It's a
fact that people who don't finish high school earn less, and
may stay on public aid longer.

You are a role model for your child. Do you want him or
her to finish high school and possibly go to college? Children watch their parents carefully from the time they're
small. If you haven't finished high school, your child may
decide graduation isn't important for him either.

It may seem hard to spend money going to school. Try to
look into the future and think of the better life an education
could provide.

After you finish high school, you may begin to see ways
of getting a college education. Sometimes an employer
pays for college tuition. Government grants and scholarships are available for women who want to go to college.

One Day at a Time

Try to take it one day at a time, and don't get too
stressed out about money worries. It helps to write down
your ideas about how you can earn more money and how
you can keep your expenses down.

In money matters, planning is important.

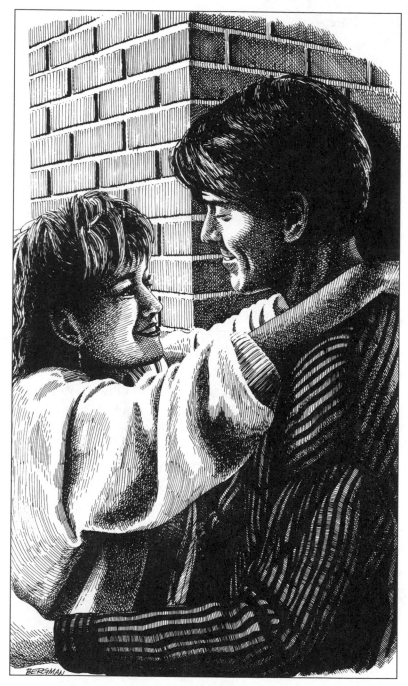

CHAPTER 10

BIRTH CONTROL MEANS LIFE CONTROL

> What if? That's crazy. It's stupid to worry.
> It hardly ever happens the first time.
> What would I do, though?
> What would become of me?
>
> Margaret Laurence—*Rachel, Rachel*

Rachel said this *after* having sex. She didn't think about the possibility of pregnancy *during* or *before* sex. Rachel, by the way, is a grown woman.

Sometimes when we feel romantic and carried away, we don't like to think about something unromantic like birth control. Sometimes it may seem like a good idea to take a chance—simply not worry about getting pregnant this time.

Why is it that in the movies nobody worries about birth control? What if you're watching a great movie, and a guy and a girl meet and are attracted to each other. In fact, they can't keep their hands off each other. Before the movie's over, they're making love.

Would it take some of the romance away if the guy said, "Excuse me, I have to put on a condom"? Or if the girl says, "I'll be right back—I have to put in my diaphragm"?

We might think, "What a slut, she planned this all along." We might think, "Oh, that's gross." Does it seem more romantic if the girl is swept away by passion for this great-looking guy, and she doesn't have to worry about something as messy and unromantic as birth control?

Real life is something like a movie. We have ideas about how scenes should be played and about how we should act. Sometimes we play these scenes in our head. Our romance scenes hardly ever have birth control in them. They usually don't have babies in them either.

Are You a Sexual Person?

We are all sexual people. How we deal with our sexuality is the issue. Some adults may be thinking that perhaps you "learned a lesson" about sex and will stay away from it until you're safely married.

Sex is a part of life. It's a natural drive. It's not like smoking (which is not natural). If you choose to be sexually active, you still have a choice about when you want another pregnancy.

After pregnancy some teens choose not to have sex again until they're older. Sometimes young women make a promise to themselves not to have sex, then find themselves lapsing again into sexual activity.

Handling Your Sexuality

In an ideal world, perhaps all girls would wait until married and then "turn on" their sexuality to become wonderfully sexy wives. This ideal world, however, is a fantasy.

Some of you will decide not to have sex for awhile because of fear of disease or another pregnancy. Maybe you don't have a partner. You may not have enjoyed sex, but engaged in it out of need for affection or cuddling. You may choose to fulfill these needs in other ways.

You have three choices. You can wait to have sex. You can have responsible (protected) sex. Or you can become pregnant again. Responsible sex means taking precautions against pregnancy and disease.

Should You Be in Love?

Sex usually is more satisfying if it's between two loving, caring people. Sex between two people who don't care for each other tends to leave one or both partners feeling worthless and ashamed. Besides, these encounters are most often spur of the moment and usually without birth control.

Some thoughts about sex:

- **Sex doesn't = love.** A young woman falls in love with someone. She believes that if she has sex with the boy, he loves her back. Sometimes people have sex for purely physical reasons, and it has nothing to do with love. Be sure that you and your partner are on the same wave length about how you feel about each other.

- **Sex can enhance a good relationship, but it cannot improve a bad one.** Sex won't make him love you more, or make him treat you right.

- **Sex is not a tool.** Sex cannot get you something else you need, like love, attention, or affection. You can get these things from a loving partner, but just

because you have sex with him doesn't mean he
will give them to you.

- **Sex is not glue.** Sex won't make him stay with you,
  or love you forever. Young men don't usually think
  of sex as a life-time bond—even if a pregnancy
  results.

- **Sex can change a relationship.** Some girls com-
  plain that once they have sex with a boy, things
  change between them. Maybe there's no challenge
  anymore, and he believes he doesn't have to take
  you out, or even be nice to you.

    If you're in a relationship like this, you are being
  used. Talk to him about how you feel about each
  other. Don't use sex as a pawn, threatening to
  withhold it, but really *talk* about what's going on in
  the relationship.

- **Don't short-change yourself sexually.** If you're
  having sex and not enjoying it, you're short-
  changing yourself. You may feel that sex is all for
  him, and you're just keeping him happy. This
  attitude leaves you feeling used and lowers your
  self-esteem.

    Every woman is capable of enjoying sex. If
  you're not, you need to talk to your partner about
  what makes you feel good and about what you
  could both do. He'll probably react enthusiastically
  about experimenting with what you both enjoy.

- **It's okay to say no.** If something is not right for
  you, or if you don't want to do it, say no. You may
  be surprised that he's relieved, too. Maybe he feels
  it's his "manly duty" to come on to you, and maybe
  he also feels it's not quite right for the two of you.

- **Unless you want another pregnancy, use birth control.**
  Nature doesn't give you "free days" when you don't have to worry about birth control. Like the first time, or the first few days after a period, or his birthday, or the day he got his first car. Mother Nature doesn't care how special the day is. She *wants* you to get pregnant to ensure that your genes are passed on.

- **Masturbation is *not* self-abuse.** Unlike some spur-of-the-moment sexual encounters (which *are* self-abuse), masturbation is a good way to release sexual urges and take the edge off sexual nervousness. Most people have done it at one time or another, so don't feel guilty, as if there's something wrong with you if you do it.

Birth Control

Statistics show that up to 15 percent of pregnant teens will become pregnant *again* within one year; 30 percent do so within two years.

Only one in three sexually active teens uses birth control (1992: *The New Teenage Body Book*). Why is this so? Here are a few reasons:

- **Some girls think, "Lightning cannot strike twice."**
  This isn't the same as lightning. Lots of girls have repeat pregnancies.

- **Birth control is not easy to get.**
  It takes planning, money, and effort. It's embarrassing to go to the clinic or doctor. Many girls say that fear and shyness prevent them from asking for birth control.

Birth control pills require follow-up visits to the doctor. Using birth control requires motivation and persistence. If money is a problem, check around for clinics that have reduced cost contraceptives.

- **"Only bad girls plan for sex."**
This is like saying, "Only good girls get pregnant." Planning for sex in order to avoid unwanted pregnancy and disease means you care about yourself and your partner.

- **Using birth control sometimes.**
Some couples use condoms "some of the time," or a girl might take the pill "sometimes." This is like playing Russian roulette. It gets tiring having to remember to take a pill every day, or to remember your diaphragm.
  Many pregnancies happen when couples "take a break" from birth control. (Remember, it's much more tiring to get up with a baby in the middle of the night.)

- **Sometimes girls get overwhelmed and give up.**
For instance, if you see yourself with no future anyway, you may think, "What's the difference if I have another baby. I have nothing else going for myself." By not using birth control, you're saying, "I don't have control over my life or anything that happens to me."

- **Other people would be unhappy if you used birth control.**
Maybe you've gotten the message that you "should have learned your lesson," or that "you won't do that again." You might be afraid that mom will find your pills or foam. It usually helps to think how mom will feel if you become pregnant again.

If you can't talk to your doctor, go to another one, or to the nearest medical clinic.

I wasn't embarrassed about talking about birth control with my boyfriend because this is my body, and I wanted to be sure I was taken care of. I think the hardest person to talk to was my mom. When I was talking to her about birth control she said, "Are you having sex with your boyfriend?"

I said, "No way."

She said she thought that giving me permission to use birth control gives me permission to have sex and she didn't want that. But kids will have sex anyway. I think if my mom could have accepted that I needed birth control, it might have been different.

Anessa, pregnant at 17

- **The same motivation that caused you to get pregnant the first time may still drive you.**
  If you feel a strong drive to create someone to love you, that drive is probably still there. If you subconsciously believed that a pregnancy would please your boyfriend, you probably still believe it. You may not consciously want to get pregnant, but the subconscious is a powerful force.

- **Magical thinking.**
  Many girls still feel that their bodies are "out of their control." Some teens say things like "Hopefully, I won't get pregnant," and "With a little luck, it won't happen again." Preventing pregnancy takes more than luck, prayer, and hope; it takes motivation and constant attention to using birth control.

- **Misinformation about birth control.**
  Some girls worry about putting a birth control

device into their body, or taking birth control pills.
Maybe you fear that it will make you infertile or
that it will make you ill. Under a doctor's care,
birth control pills are safe and reliable (when taken
every day).

For the few who cannot take the pill, other
reliable methods are available. Fertility almost
always returns when you stop taking the pill or
using the device.

*It's the woman's responsibility to use contracep-
tives. You can't depend on the guy. If you're going to
be sexually active, you must take the responsibility.
It's fine to talk about condoms, but he may not have
one. And you're the one who will have to support this
child, and the best way you can do it is get yourself on
some kind of birth control and be responsible for it.*

*You can't take it lightly, just as you can't take the
care of your child lightly. You don't want your child
outside in the street in the cold with no shoes or socks.
That's not being responsible.*

*You have to look at the pill in the same way. Every
morning I'm going to take this pill. I'm going to see a
doctor and I'm going to take care of myself. You can't
be careless about it because having another baby is a
big responsibility.*

Jobita, 16, mother of Ericel, 2

Risk of AIDS

Jobita is right—as far as she goes. It is the woman's
responsibility to use birth control. But it is also the man's.
The pill won't protect you from STDs or HIV. Every time
you have sex, the man needs to use a condom—to protect
both of you. You can carry one in your purse if you think

he might not have one. Getting pregnant when you aren't ready is not very responsible. Getting AIDS is much worse, and only the condom protects you from AIDS. And of course, using a condom means you're practicing "safer sex." Nothing, not even a condom, will absolutely protect you from AIDS—except abstinence.

To get control of your life, you decide when you want another child. If you want one right away, then you don't need to worry about birth control.

If you don't, you can find a birth control method that works for you. The chart on page 150 shows the different birth control methods.

These Won't Prevent Pregnancy

- **Having sex during your period.**
  You could ovulate during your period.

- **Breastfeeding.**
  You could ovulate even though you're breast-feeding your baby.

- **Douching.**
  Many girls try douching with various things—soda pop, vinegar, douche, water. Douching isn't a birth control method. It may even provide an additional stream of fluid to force the sperm into the uterus.

- **Vaginal hygiene sprays.**
  Don't confuse these with contraceptives.

- **Not having an orgasm.**
  Your orgasm has little to do with getting pregnant.

- **Going to the bathroom right after sex.**
  Those sperm are too fast for this to help.

- **Jumping up and down afterward.**
  You're wasting your energy.

RELIABLE BIRTH CONTROL METHODS

Method	Doctor's visit?	Effective?	Advantages	Disadvantages
The Pill	Yes	99%	Easy to use. Doesn't interrupt lovemaking. May help regulate periods.	Causes side effects for some. Must take a pill every day. No protection against AIDS, other STDs.
Diaphragm, Cervical cap	Yes, must be fitted.	90-95%	No side effects. Low cost.	Must be used every time you have sex. No protection against AIDS, other STDs.
Condom for men; Condom for women	No. Can buy in drugstores, vending machines	90%.	No side effects. One method male can use. Protects against STDs, AIDS.	Some people don't like the way they feel. Sometimes break or leak. Use with jelly or foam. May interrupt lovemaking.
Foam, Sponge	No. Can buy in various places.	70-90%.	Can be used when needed.	Higher risk of pregnancy. May interrupt lovemaking. Can be messy.
Norplant	Yes. Hormone implants put in arm.	99%	No planning before lovemaking. Lasts five years.	Cost may be prohibitive. Irregular periods. No protection against AIDS, other STDs.
IUD	Yes	96-98%	Doesn't interrupt lovemaking. Lasts up to 10 years.	Possible cramps, heavy menstrual flow. Increased risk of pelvic inflammatory disease (PID). No protection against AIDS, STDs.
Depo-Provera	Yes	99.7%	Doesn't interrupt lovemaking. Lasts 3 months.	Possible side effects such as irregular menstrual bleeding at first. Must get injection every 3 months. No protection against AIDS, other STDs.

- **Withdrawal, or not inserting the penis fully into the vagina.**
  Some girls have gotten pregnant through panties or without insertion. Sperm are strong swimmers and very motivated creatures.

- **Taking one or several birth control pills before having intercourse.**
  Some girls borrow someone else's pills and take one or more from a packet. Chances are both girls will get pregnant. Birth control pills have to be taken every day to be effective.

  In fact, *the pill is not an effective contraceptive during the first month you take it.* You need to use another form of contraceptive until you've been on the pill for a month

- **Standing up to have sex.**
  Gravity doesn't have anything to do with it. Sperm can swim uphill.

- **Home-made birth control devices.**
  Plastic wrap, balloons used like a condom, or regular sponges do not work as birth control devices.

- **Wishful thinking.**
  That's all it is.

Sex Isn't Always Planned

Let's say that it's a year from now. You decided after your baby's birth that you'd wait until marriage to have sex. Your boyfriend disappeared soon after you told him you were pregnant.

You're feeling alone and miserable. The baby keeps you up most nights (even though he's a year old).

An old friend invites you to a party. You go and have the best time you've had in a long time. You feel free and happy. You feel sexy. You have too much to drink. Your old friend hugs you and kisses you. You feel more loved than you have in a long time. You don't care about tomorrow. You don't care about yesterday. One thing leads to another and you have sex.

Now, it's the next day. How do you feel? Are you scared? You start counting the days since your last period. You're a little relieved that it wasn't right in the middle of your cycle, but you're still not sure. What if you're pregnant again? You promise never to have sex again.

Infrequent sex is a problem for lots of young girls. It's hard to plan for birth control when you haven't planned for sex. It's understandable that you wouldn't want to be on the pill *all* the time if you're only having sex occasionally.

It's good to be prepared with some barrier method, like condoms and foam, or a contraceptive sponge. Then, if you get into a regular relationship, you can change methods if you like.

Remember, only a condom helps protect you against AIDS. Next to abstinence, you are safest if the man uses a condom and the woman, contraceptive foam. That way, your chances of protecting both of you from pregnancy and AIDS are fairly good.

If he won't use a condom, will you use a female condom? Or will you abstain from sex? Your only other choice is to risk getting HIV which leads to AIDS.

Making Birth Control Work

Motivation and *persistence* make birth control work. Motivation is simply having the *desire* to postpone another pregnancy until you and your partner are ready and able to love and care for a child. Some girls, however, may not have a strong desire to avoid pregnancy. It's good to know how you feel about pregnancy, so you can make a choice.

I take birth control pills, and I make sure I take them. Even my boyfriend reminds me because I don't want any more babies right now.

I have friends who aren't taking birth control, and all they will say is that they're just not. I don't understand that because I learned. Maybe they just want another baby—if you aren't on anything, you're going to get pregnant whether it's a month or a year later. You may think you'll be lucky, but you won't be.

Frederica, 15, mother of Elias, 5 months

Day to day persistence and foresight are required to make birth control work. If you want to prevent pregnancy, this means getting into the habit of using birth control when you have sexual intercourse. Here's an exercise to help you with motivation:

1) Get comfortable, sit in a chair with your arms by your side.

2) Close your eyes.

3) Imagine yourself two years in the future. Where are you? What are you doing? Imagine that you're pregnant again. How do you feel about it?

4) Open your eyes. Are you relieved that you're not pregnant again?

Many girls feel that it's unfair when they become pregnant. After all, lots of girls have sex and *they* don't get pregnant. Remember that it's not an accident if you don't use birth control and get pregnant. In fact, if you don't use protection, it's an accident if you *don't* get pregnant!

Four out of five young women will get pregnant within a year if they have sex without birth control.

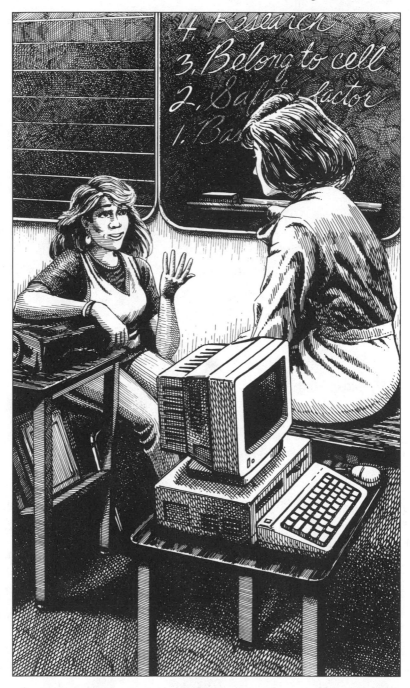

CHAPTER 11

GETTING WHAT YOU WANT

What I want now is different than before I had the baby. Before, I didn't really have any goals. I was working at a fast-food place and thinking that was fine. Now, with Sean, I've started to want more for us.

Terry, 16, mother of Sean, 8 months

I want to graduate, get a job, and move into a better district. The kids around here don't respect their parents, and I don't want Felipe to grow up here. There are too many troubles, little kids writing on the walls, breaking holes in the fences. I don't want Felipe doing these things. There are too many fights, too many people shooting each other here.

I want a job, but if I start working now, I won't go back to school. I can get a better job if I graduate.

Maria 15, mother of Felipe, 2

Some people seem to know from the time they are small children what they want to be, what they want to do in life. Sometimes having a baby changes what we want for ourselves. Sometimes we don't know where we want our lives to go.

Donna has a new baby, and for now, she's wrapped up in the daily care of her baby. She says, "I don't know what I want. We just go day by day."

As time goes on, Donna will probably start to think about what she wants for herself and her baby.

A Job Can Build Self-Esteem

Some young women want to stay home with their children. They may have enough outside support to do that. Others, however, find their self-esteem suffers when they stay home:

I think staying home is a difficult thing for any mother to do. I think that was the worst three months of my life—staying home and living on welfare.

It was between college and going to work. The doctor prescribed Prozac because I couldn't handle staying home. I can stay home one day from work, and I'm dying to go back the very next day.

Working mothers should remember it's the quality, not the quantity of mothering. You could be home all day with your kids and spend no time with them—and you can go to work and come home and spend one good hour together.

Amy, 23, mother of Kent, 7

Parents who continue their education get better jobs and usually do better through life than those who don't. Their children also do better through their lives because they follow their parent's example.

Having a good job makes you feel good about yourself.

My being happy has so much to do with mothering.
When I was depressed, I couldn't get into mothering
Rudy and Joy like I wanted to. I would try to force
myself, but I couldn't. Then I would feel guilty.

The kids and I had a rough life for about a year
after I split. I had realized I didn't love Ellis, that
I never did. I didn't love him, but I needed him—
I don't know why. He was never working, and I was
miserable with him. I was on welfare almost the entire
time. I was so miserable that I hated myself and
I hated him.

Then I started getting stronger. I finally moved into
an apartment by myself.

When I went to school to be a medical assistant, I
felt so good because I knew I was doing something for
me. I wanted something in medicine, but I wanted to
do it quickly. I have gotten into a field I love, one I've
wanted to be in ever since I was a little girl.

That's important. You have got to do things for
yourself, you have got to be happy with yourself
before you can be happy with your kids.

Brigette, 22, mother of Rudy, 3, and Joy, 4

As Brigette found out, it *is* important to like your work.
If you hate your work, move on to something better:

I tried working in a factory, and there's nothing
there except hard work. If you know a skill like com-
puter skills, you can get into business jobs where you
don't have to work so hard, get so dirty. I think
everyone should at least take a computer course. A lot
of people don't like it, but if you can use a computer,
you can always find a job.

Shelley, 20, mother of Virginia, 4

Of course, if you hate working with computers, that's not the answer for you. You have many other choices.

What Can You Be?

There are lots of different jobs and careers. Maybe you know that you'd like to make money, but you don't know how you want to do that. You might not know what's available to you. Your school counselor could help you know what's out there. Here are some examples of careers:

- **Do you like to help people?**
  Doctor or nurse
  Social worker
  Counselor
  Teacher
  Childcare worker

- **Do you want to work in an office?**
  Bank clerk
  Accountant or bookkeeper
  Administrative Assistant
  Business Manager

- **Do you like to work outside?**
  Landscaping
  Pool maintenance
  Forestry Service
  Carpenter

- **Do you want to create something?**
  Construction worker
  Caterer or cook
  Floral designer

- **Do you like technology?**
  Computer programmer
  Computer operator or data entry operator
  Electronics technician

These are just a few examples. There are many more. It might help to write down some ideas about what you want to be. Look at jobs that women don't ordinarily choose, like plumbing or carpentry. If you like them, they can pay well.

Choose something that interests you. One way to figure this out is to write down your interests. Then, find out what jobs fit those interests. If you're not in school, or if your school counselor can't help you, is there a college near you? Perhaps they have a Women's Center designed to help mothers and other women with career planning.

Education Is Important

Education is a good way for women to increase their earning power. If you're going to work anyway, why not make as much as you can and be in a job you enjoy?

People say, "Oh, you have a baby—I guess you dropped out of school."

I say, "No, she didn't stop me from going to school. I'm going to graduate with my class." I like school now. After I graduate, I'm going on to college.

Candi, 16, Janet, 18 months

You may be tempted to wait until the baby is older or until things settle down before you go back to school. It's much easier to continue your education rather than stopping and going back. Many of those who wait never go back.

After I graduated, I was thinking about not going on to school for a couple of years. Then I thought, if I work for two years, I won't go back. So I decided to go on right now. I'll start getting my training soon to be an RN. I'd like to work in an emergency room or with patients coming out of surgery.

Ginny, 17, mother of Juan, 4 months

You have to take the chance if you want to get
ahead. I used to say, "Well, I'll start school, but if it
gets too involved, I'll just quit." Now I'm thinking
about the better future I'll have if I get an education.

In September I'm going back to school in the
evening. If that doesn't work, I may quit working, get
a grant, and go to school full-time. I think I'll put my
school first now.

Often I think, "Oh, I have to work," but I want to
get ahead. Administration of justice—counseling—
something to do with the police force but not out on
the street. I always wanted to be a probation officer.

Shelley

It gets exciting to think that you can decide what you
want to do and then get the education to do it. It may seem
too hard at times, but when you look at it in smaller steps, it
won't seem so hard.

Four Steps To What You Want
Step 1: Find a role model.

A role model is someone who has done what you want to
do. It's nice if the role model is someone you know, but it
doesn't have to be. S/he can be someone you admire and
look up to.

A role model could be a business woman in your community, your teacher, or your counselor. A role model can
also be a young man or woman your own age who is doing
what you want to do.

Some of the best role models "live" in your local library.
The library has books on any subject that interests you.
You'll find biographies and audio tapes.

If your role model is someone you can talk to, approach
that person to see if s/he'd be willing to "mentor" you. A

mentor is a teacher/leader. You may be surprised at that person's willingness to help.

The first and biggest step you can take toward getting what you want is: **Ask for advice from someone who can help you.**

Step 2: Set goals.

Goals are like stairsteps. Imagine the thing you want at the top of the stairs. Suppose your goal is to finish high school. What steps do you need to take to finish high school?

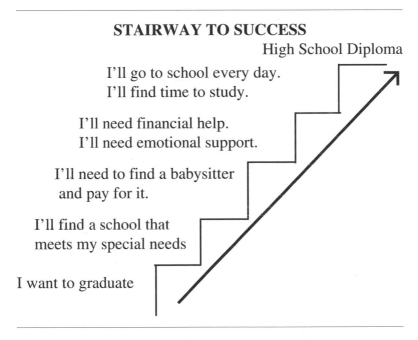

STAIRWAY TO SUCCESS

High School Diploma

I'll go to school every day.
I'll find time to study.

I'll need financial help.
I'll need emotional support.

I'll need to find a babysitter
and pay for it.

I'll find a school that
meets my special needs

I want to graduate

Breaking down your goals this way helps you see the steps you must take to get to your final goal. You'll get a feeling of accomplishment as you reach each goal. It's good to set a time limit on when you'll get what you want. What happens if you don't make it? You change the deadline, but it gives you something to shoot for. It's a

good idea to reward yourself in some way after each step
is completed.

You can have more than one goal ladder. Some of your
goals may not be related, so the steps you take are on
different ladders. For instance, you can have *career* goals
and *social* goals. Maybe you want a career, but you also
want to have good friends. You may do different things to
get to each goal.

You'll find, though, that as you meet some goals, the
others follow. As you work toward your career goals, you
may make some wonderful friends.

Some Tips About Setting Goals:

- Give your goals definite deadlines.

- Make your goals clear and specific.

- Make sure your goals are realistic.

- Review your goals often.

- Use your goals to get through tough times.

- Tell your goals to people who care.

Step 3: Define the steps to get to your goal.

How do you get to each rung on the ladder? It helps to
know the things to do and the choices to make along the
way. You may already have an idea about what you need to
do to get to each step on your ladder. If you're not sure,
your role model can help you list those things, or you can
do more thinking about your goal.

You may have to be creative to take some of these steps.
For instance, suppose you want to finish high school and
eventually go on to college. Maybe you know how to do
the first step—finish high school. Break down the activities
you need to do to finish high school. There might be more
activities than you thought.

Is childcare the problem? Do you have to work and go to

school at the same time? It helps to write down these
problems and solve them one at a time.

Step 4: Compare your results with your goals.

Sometimes we have to make tough choices. Maybe
you're trying to work *and* go to school. What if your boss
decides to make you work longer hours and you don't have
any more hours to give? You must make a choice. Should
you work longer hours (maybe for more pay) or find a less
demanding job and continue school?

It's helpful to think about a few years from now or even
a year from now. If you give up this job, will you be sorry
one year from now? Will you be better off finishing high
school and trying for college? There's probably another job
like the one you'd give up. There's probably a *better* one.

It helps to revise your goals when necessary and to give
yourself a little more time. Remind yourself of your goals
when you're confused about what choices to make. Never
make a choice that makes it harder for you to reach your
goal. Remember to reward yourself as you achieve
each goal.

Sometimes You Need a Little Help

Sometimes you *do* need outside help. Childcare is likely
to be a problem. Try calling your local Social Services or
United Way. Maybe there's a teen mom program with an
infant center in your area.

Money may also be a problem. There is an old proverb
that goes: "Give a man a fish, he eats for a day; teach a man
to fish, he eats for a lifetime." Accept any help available to
you as long as it "teaches you to fish" and as long as it
doesn't take away from your self-esteem. Check out government programs and grants to assist you financially while
going to school. Check with your local Social Services
Department.

Sometimes family members are willing and able to help while you're working on your goals. Remember to check with more than one place. After you graduate from high school, you may decide you want to go to college or trade school. Some people put themselves through college with a lot of small grants and loans.

When applying for jobs, it's a good idea to ask about education benefits. Many companies will pay for your college while you work. Some even pay for things like books and parking while you're going to school.

Take On the Challenge

It's not always bad when people tell you that you can't do something. Some girls take it as a personal challenge:

> *My real reason I'm trying so hard is because my mother's family downed me for having the baby, saying I'm nothing but a tramp. Nobody on that side thinks I'll finish school. They think I'll have two or three more kids before I'm out of school. I want to do it for myself—but also to prove something to them. I want to be somebody.*
>
> Melanie, 15, mother of Alice, 13 months

> *I was going to stay home until after I had the baby, but when I heard of the special class, I decided to go back to school. I might never have finished high school except my older sister always said I'd be the one who would drop out. I decided to show her.*
>
> Alta, 22, mother of Howard, 3, and Marta, 6

Perhaps your boyfriend or husband is threatened by the thought of you getting an education or working. Maybe he's afraid that you'll meet someone else, or that you'll be better educated than he is:

*My husband doesn't want me to go back to school,
but I want to. I tell him we need me to work because
of inflation and everything. If he insists, I don't know
what I'll do. I'll try to convince him. He only went
through sixth grade, but his father taught him to drive
tractors, and he's a good mechanic.*

Deanna, 15, mother of Paula, 3 weeks

If your boyfriend or husband is discouraging you from
building your future, try talking to him about his fears.
Maybe you can get him to see that you'd be helping *his*
future, too. If you can get him to talk about the things that
threaten him, you may be able to convince him that you're
simply trying to help all of you, just as he is.

Get Started on Your Future

It's tough sometimes to keep pushing forward. Sometimes it seems easier to quit. When you're riding a bicycle
up a hill, it's hard work—until you get to the top. Then,
you can stop at the top, look around a little, and start down
the other side. That's much like working on your goals. If
you keep making progress, you'll be there before you
know it.

What happens when you get there? Usually, you'll set
bigger goals.

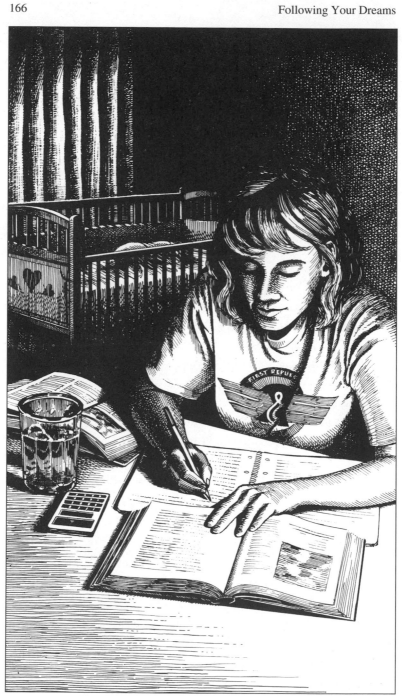

CHAPTER 12

FOLLOWING
YOUR DREAMS

People may say that the odds are against you. You might hear that you'll probably live in poverty, be dependent on other people, and that your life script has already been written for you.

The fact is, you can be in charge of writing your life script if you want to. You can grow your own garden instead of waiting for someone to give you flowers.

Despite the odds against them, many women have survived teen pregnancy and have gone on to live out their dreams, to raise families, to have successful marriages, and to have good careers. Some are well-known.

Oprah Winfrey was pregnant at fourteen, and she went on to become a talented actress and host of her own talk show. Roseanne Barr presented adoptive parents with a daughter when she was in her late teens. She went on to

become a comedienne and star. Whoopie Goldberg, herself
a single parent, has helped her daughter deal with a teen
pregnancy.

You may not recognize the names of most teen moms,
but you understand their experiences. It isn't easy though,
as one teen mom understands:

> *It's hard to parent on your own. If I had to do it
> again, I wouldn't. I would do it really different be-
> cause I still want to run around and do my own thing.*
>
> *When I go shopping, the baby goes with me. On the
> weekends I spend mornings and afternoons with him.
> Sometimes I go out on Friday and Saturday nights. I
> spend week nights with him, but soon I'll start a class.*
>
> *When people tell you it's going to be difficult,
> believe them. It's going to be a lot harder than they
> say it is. I knew it would be a hassle, but I didn't think
> it would be as hard as it is being a full-time mother
> and going to work.*
>
> *I'll start college in the fall, but that will be only for
> a couple of years. Then it will be easier. It's going to
> get harder before it gets easier because I have a lot to
> do to prepare my life for both of us.*
>
> *I have to be able to support myself and the baby by
> myself before I go ahead and get married. I don't
> want to be stuck with no education and no job skills. I
> want Gary to have the best there is.*
>
> Leica, 18, mother of Gary, 3 months

The Joy of Making Choices

In the movie, "The Little Mermaid," Ariel is a teenage
mermaid who has dreams of breaking away from her
undersea world. To us, her world seems like a magical
place full of bright colors and pretty sounds. To Ariel, the
human world is magical, and she longs to be part of it.

Against her father's wishes, Ariel falls in love with a human. She makes the choice to leave her colorful world and become part of a world that seems harsh and dangerous to her father.

Ariel's choices seem strange and different to her family and friends, but she makes the choices that feel right to her, and she is happy. Once she makes her choice, forces come to her aid to help her accomplish her goals and find the happiness she seeks.

We don't know if Ariel's choice will *always* make her happy. She may feel a little sadness at times for things left behind, but we know that she feels joy for having made her own decisions and set her own direction.

Some girls believe that to really make it in the outside world, they'll need a husband to help them. Marriage works out great for some, but girls who *don't* get married young tend to do better:

I'm trying to think more about myself now. I think a lot of girls get into a situation where they don't think highly of themselves. For a long time I stuck with Ben because I thought that was what I deserved. Finally I realized—why should I be taking this when I haven't done anything wrong?

We thought our role was me and him and the baby, and eventually we were supposed to get married. I think I would have put myself real low as a person if I had gone on. Neither one of us was happy. I finally realized we couldn't keep something we had five years ago. I would think, we used to do this, we used to do that—but that's what we used to do, not what is happening now. Now is what is important.

We loved each other. I guess we still do because we were each the first love of the other. It's sad, but I'm happy now. I understand why a lot of girls are on

welfare when they're young, but I think they should
try moving on.
    A woman shouldn't try to stay in the same place.
She should try to make herself a better place. The only
way you can be happy is if you have respect for
yourself.

Shelley, 20, mother of Virginia, 4

Shelley knows that she has to grow and become self-reliant herself before she can become part of a couple. She knows that another person can't *make* her happy—she has to find her own happiness.

Tools to Help You

Since you're young, you have a long time to work on your goals and your future. You don't have to do it overnight. You *do* have to know what to work toward and how far you want to go.

Give some real thought to what you want to do with your life, what you want to be. Making goals and following through with them will make you self-confident.

There are things you can do every day to make your life a little easier. Staying in school, or going back to school is one of the biggest steps you can take to improve your chances.

All of us have times when we feel emotions such as jealousy, anger, and frustration. You might already have your own ways of dealing with these emotions. You may enjoy exercise, curling up with a book or movie, calling friends and talking, or just being alone for a while.

One of the fastest ways to change your mood is to change your posture and your breathing. When you're depressed you probably slump a little, hold your head down, and your breathing is shallow. Sitting or standing tall, breathing deeply, and looking up will probably make you feel better immediately.

There are other tricks you can use to get out of negative moods and into positive resourceful ones as quickly as possible. Here are a few tools:

Meditation

Meditation is a way to help manage stress. Meditation means giving yourself a few minutes a day to relax, close your eyes, go "into yourself," and stop thinking about your problems. It gives your mind a little rest. You can do it in a few minutes every day. You can choose a certain time of the day to spend a few minutes meditating, or you can do it when you feel the need to relax.

1) Go to a quiet place or play some soft, relaxing music.

2) Close your eyes, relax, and take long, deep breaths.

3) Clear your mind. Try to let your mind float to a far-away place. The place should be beautiful and comfortable. Maybe it's a place in the mountains or on the beach where you're by yourself and totally relaxed and at peace.

4) Stay in your peaceful spot until you feel relaxed and rested.

5) Toward the end of your meditation session, try telling yourself something positive. For instance, tell yourself that you're strong, intelligent, and capable, and you know you'll make it through this stressful time.

Meditation is a time to let your imagination go. Imagine what it would be like to have what you want in life. When you're ready to be Steven Spielberg, you can turn these thoughts into movies!

Movies for the Mind

Have you ever noticed that sometimes when you're not feeling so good about yourself, your mind drags out old memories of bad times and relives them? My sister and I recently talked about a childhood experience that we had. She remembered it in an entirely different way than I did. Our minds store the things that happen to us, but they may choose to make some things larger or smaller, or more or less important.

So, you have movies stored in your brain of things that have happened to you, and you can play them back whenever you want. But, did you know that you can change these movies? You can learn to replay them so that you have more control over how they end. You can play the movie as fast as you want, or you can stop it. You can make new movies of your past.

You can also make a movie of your future, step into it, and feel how it would be. This makes your future seem more real, and you will be in control. It helps your mind set a course for what you want.

See Your Past Differently

Is there something in your past that you feel controls the things you do now? Maybe you regret something you did. Maybe you have a fear of trying a new relationship. Or, maybe you haven't forgotten something that someone did to you.

In order to get on with the future, we usually need to put our past behind us. This exercise won't change what has happened to you during your life, but it will help control how you feel about it now.

1) Go to a comfortable place, sit down or lie down, and close your eyes. Now, pretend that you are a

projectionist in a movie theater. Think of the time in your past that used to cause you pain or control your life. You're going to run a black and white movie of this event. As you imagine yourself standing at a comfortable distance from the screen, watch the movie.

2) Let the movie play on the screen of your mind. You can stop the movie at any point that you feel uncomfortable. You can run it backwards, or change speeds to very fast or slow motion. This helps you realize that *you* are in control.

   Then, start the film forward again until you get past the painful point. You can do this as many times as you need to.

3) Try adding music, either your favorite music (you can really play it if you'd like) or silly music, like circus tunes or skating-rink tunes. Doing this means you can change how close you are to the movie, or how far away. Take time to notice how you feel.

4) You can change what people say in your movie. Maybe you wanted to do something different or say something different. You can do that in your movie. You can change what someone else said to you.

Picturing Your Future

You can use the same movie tool to visualize your future. Doing this helps you see the kind of future you'd like to have. Playing a movie of your future helps you believe that it's possible.

1) Choose something in the future that you want for yourself, or how you want to be in the future. It should be something *good*. It should be something that you really want.

2) Like a movie director, create a movie of yourself in the future getting what you want. This movie will be in color. Let the movie play in your mind. Now step into the movie.

   You'll feel like you're there instead of watching from a distance. How do you feel as the good things happen to you? What do you see? What do you feel? What do you hear?

   What are the people in the movie doing? Make the color seem brighter.

3) Store this movie away in your mind to use when needed. Or, you can change the movies whenever you want. Whenever you need it, close your eyes and "see" the good movie.

You can do whatever you want in these movies. If the movie is about something you need to put behind you, you'll watch the movie from a distance. If the movie is about something you want for your future, you'll imagine seeing yourself *in* the movie.

Self-Talk

Another great way to change your future is by changing not only your movies, but also what you say to yourself.

People remember and believe 70 percent of what they say to themselves. Most of us talk to ourselves. Sometimes we say things to ourselves that we'd never say to a friend (or even an enemy). Self-talk can build you up instead of tearing you down.

You may have to retrain yourself to say positive things. At first it may take a lot of effort because you'll have to relearn the way you talk to yourself. The way you talk to yourself becomes a habit, and habits can be changed.

1) Be aware of the way you're thinking. Are you thinking, "I feel okay now, but it won't last"? Try changing the thought to, "I feel okay, and I can feel this way more and more of the time."

2) Stand in front of the mirror and say, "You know, there are a lot of things about you that I like." Go on to tell yourself what you like about yourself. It's better if you say it out loud, but saying it in your mind works, too. You can use the time you're brushing your teeth or doing your hair to do this. If you can't find anything nice to say to yourself, just say, "I love you."

3) If you find that your mind is straying to something that upsets you, say "Stop." If you catch yourself saying *anything* negative to yourself (even if you think it's true), yell "Stop" in your mind. Say something to yourself that makes you feel happy or proud, even if it's a future thing. Something like, "I *am* going to finish high school."

4) If you're upset, try doing the self-talk while doing something physical. Take a walk, a bicycle ride, or do aerobics or other exercises, for example. This will get rid of some of the energy built up from being upset.

   While you're walking, send some positive messages to yourself. Since you're upset, they might be things to calm you. For instance, you might say, "I'm all right. I'll work everything out."

You've Been Given a Challenge

I've heard people call teen pregnancy a "tragedy," a "mistake," and a "shame." I have come to think of it as a challenge and an opportunity. It's a challenge of choice.

You now have the opportunity to make choices for your future and for your baby's future. You have the challenge of setting goals for yourself and finding ways to make them happen. You have the challenge of asking others for help when you need it. You have the opportunity to teach other young women what you've learned.

If I could do it again, what would I do differently? I'd probably finish school faster. I'd work on my goals with more energy. For a while I believed what everyone else believed, that teen moms usually don't finish high school, and that they usually live in poverty. What matters is what *you* believe.

If I could do it again, I'd reach out sooner to other teen mothers. You can help each other, and you can help other young teenagers struggling with questions about sex and self-esteem.

If I could do it again, I wouldn't feel guilty about choices I made for myself and my daughter. Some choices seem selfish on the surface, but they help you in the long run—spending time and money on going to college, for instance.

If I could do it again, I wouldn't be afraid to ask for help when I needed it. Every young mother needs help with money, childcare, and emotional problems. Don't be afraid to ask.

Through the years I've realized that the challenge of teen pregnancy has been my greatest teacher. I've learned about asking for and accepting help when I needed it, about daring to dream beyond what others thought I deserved, and about reaching out to others who need help.

Accept the challenge to go as far as you can go. If you make a good effort to keep you and your baby healthy, to ask for help when you need it, to set goals for yourself, and always to try to make positive choices, you'll build a good future for you and your baby. You'll make mistakes along the way—I did—but you'll make lots of *good* choices too.

How Do You Know When You're "There"?

You won't look out your window one day and see that a garden has magically appeared. You'll plant the seeds and water it and give it sunshine and let it grow. You'll gradually notice that you're becoming more self-reliant. You'll notice that things are working out for you and that you have more and more opportunities coming your way.

You'll look out your window and see a garden, but you won't be surprised, because *you* made it grow.

I have faith in you. *You are a survivor.*

Appendix

Bibliography

Barr, Linda, and Catherine Monserrat. *Teenage Pregnancy: A New Beginning.* 1991. New Futures, Inc., 5400 Cutler, NE, Albuquerque, NM 87110.

Prenatal health book written specifically for pregnant adolescents.

Bingham, Mindy, and Sandy Stryker. *Career Choices and Changes: A Guide for Teens and Young Adults.* 1994. 304 pp. Academic Innovations, 3463 State Street, Suite 219, Santa Barbara, CA 93105. 804/967-8015.

This book provides an activity-oriented approach to career decision-making that helps teens discover their unique interests and talents. Who am I? What do I want? How do I get it?

Brinkley, Ginny, and Sherry Sampson. *Young and Pregnant—A Book for You.* 1989. 73 pp. Pink Inc!, P.O. Box 866, Atlantic Beach, FL 32233-0866. 904/2885-9276.

Refreshingly simple book on prenatal care directed to teenagers. Provides basic information. Also see *You and Your New Baby: A Book for Young Mothers,* same authors. Both titles available in Spanish.

Eggebroten, Anne, Ed. *Abortion, My Choice, God's Grace: Christian Women Tell Their Stories.* 1994. 238 pp. New Paradigm Books, P.O. Box 60008, Pasadena, CA 91116.

Moving first-person accounts which "confront the reality of abortion as a morally responsible choice made by countless Christian women, including many from the most conservative traditions," Theological implications are discussed which can help a young woman make the best decision for herself.

Fenwick, Elizabeth, and Richard Walker. *How Sex Works.* 1994. 96 pp. Dorling Kindersley Publishing, Inc., 95 Madison Avenue, New York, NY 10016.

For teenagers. Profusely illustrated, easy-to-read guide to emotional, physical, and sexual maturity. Includes quotes from teens.

Gilman, Lois. *The Adoption Resource Book.* 1992. 400 pp. HarperCollins Publishers, Inc., 10 East 53rd Street, New York, NY 10022-5299. 212/207-7000.

Comprehensive guide to adoption is aimed at potential adoptive parents. Includes positive descriptions of independent as well as agency adoption. Also included is a brief account of open adoption and the advantages associated with openness.

Hamilton-Wilkes, Donald L. and Viola. *Teen Guide—Job Search: 10 Easy Steps to Your Future.* 1993. 112 pp. JEM/JOB Educational Materials, 1230 E. Main St., Alhambra, CA 91801. 818/308-7642.

Simplified, practical, basic approach to job hunting. Excellent for teens beginning their job search. Good resource.

Heine, Arthur J. *Surviving After High School: Overcoming Life's Hurdles.* 1991. 240 pp. J-Mart Press. Order from Keller-Huff Training and Consulting, R.R. 2, Box 276, Highway 100, Hermann, MO 65041. 314/486-5348.

Contains *lots* of information about independent living—
getting and keeping a job, taxes, budgets, shopping, handling a
checking account and credit card, housing, transportation, and
much more.

Johnson, Joy and Dr. S. M., et al. *Pregnant, This Time It's
Me.* 1992. 24 pp. Centering Corporation, 1531 N.
Saddlecreek Road, Omaha, NE 68104 5064.

Simply written booklet of advice for pregnant teens.

Kuklin, Susan. *What Do I Do Now?* 1991. 142 pp. Putnam
Publishing Group, 200 Madison Avenue, New
York, NY 10016. 800/631-8571.

Based on interviews with pregnant teens. Includes accounts of
adoption, abortion, and keeping the baby, and suggests no
easy answers for too-early pregnancy.

Lindsay, Jeanne Warren. *Do I Have a Daddy? A Story
About a Single-Parent Child.* Illustrated by Cheryl
Boller. 1991. Morning Glory Press, Inc., 6595 San
Haroldo Way, Buena Park, CA 90620.

This is a picture book/story in which a single mother explains
to her son that his daddy left soon after he was born. It
contains a 12-page section of suggestions for single parents
facing the question, "Do I have a daddy?"

_____. *Parents, Pregnant Teens and the Adoption
Option: Help for Families.* 1989. 208 pp. Morning
Glory Press.

Based on interviews with parents of pregnant teens considering an adoption plan. Helps parents understand that, while
adoption may be a good decision, it is never easy for the
extended family *or* the birthparents.

_____. *School-Age Parents: The Challenge of Three-
Generation Living.* 1990. 224 pp. Morning Glory.

A much needed book for dealing with the frustrations,
problems, and pleasures of three-generation living. A must for

pregnant and parenting teens and their families. Deals with emotional as well as practical issues. Many quotes from teens and their parents.

_____. *Teenage Couples—Caring, Commitment, and Change. Teenage Couples—Coping with Reality.* 1995. 208, 192 pp. Morning Glory Press, Inc.

Two books on relationships for teenagers. Based on in-depth interviews with teen couples and on nationwide survey of more than three thousand teenagers' attitudes toward marriage. Realistic and helpful. See also *Teenage Couples— Expectations and Reality,* an account of the research behind the two books written for teens.

_____. *Teens Parenting—Your Baby's First Year. Teens Parenting—The Challenge of Toddlers.* 1991. 192 pp. each. Morning Glory Press, Inc.

Two how-to-parent books especially for teenage parents. Ages and stages from one month to three years are described along with the unique needs of children at each stage.

_____. *Teen Dads: Rights, Responsibilities, and Joys.* 1993. 192 pp. Morning Glory Press, Inc.

A guide for teen fathers who want to develop their parenting skills, with emphasis on dealing with children from birth to the age of three, and on the father's role during pregnancy. For fathers, whether they live with child or not.

_____ and Jean Brunelli, PHN. *Teens Parenting: Your Pregnancy and Newborn Journey.* 1994. 192 pp. Morning Glory Press, Inc.

Prenatal health care written to special needs of pregnant teens. Fetal development, prenatal nutrition, discomforts of pregnancy, labor and delivery, the adoption option, appearance and care of the newborn, infant feeding, and the mother's "fourth trimester" are discussed. One chapter focuses on the father of the baby. Also available in Spanish edition.

Marecek, Mary. *Breaking Free from Partner Abuse.* 1993. 96 pp. Morning Glory Press.

Underlying message is that the reader does not deserve to be hit. Simply written. Can help a young woman escape an abusive relationship.

Mathes, Patricia G., and Beverly J. Irby. *Teen Pregnancy and Parenting Handbook.* 1993. 430 pp. Research Press, 2612 North Mattis Avenue, Champaign, IL 61821.

Very detailed book about reproduction, pregnancy, labor and delivery, sexuality, and parenting through the first year.

McCoy, Kathy, and Charles Wibbelsman, M.D. *The Teen-age Body Book Guide.* 1992. The Putnam Publishing Group, 200 Madison Avenue, New York, NY 10016.

This is a book crammed with information for teenagers about everything from their bodies, changing feelings, teenage beauty, and special medical needs of young adults to sexuality, venereal disease, birth control, pregnancy and parenthood. The book is written directly to teenagers. Lots of quotes from young people, sometimes in the form of questions, are included in each chapter.

Miller, Kathryn Ann. *Did My First Mother Love Me?* 1994. 48 pp. Morning Glory Press.

A wonderful story for every adopted child who wonders about his/her birthparents. Written by a birthmother as a letter to her child.

Reynolds, Marilyn. *Detour for Emmy.* 1993. 256 pp. *Too Soon for Jeff.* 1994. 224 pp. Morning Glory Press.

Two wonderfully absorbing novels about teenage pregnancy. Emmy has a baby at 15 and finds her life changing drastically. Jeff is a reluctant teenage father who eventually decides to share responsibility for his son.

Sander, Joelle. *Before Their Time: Four Generations of Teenage Mothers.* 1991. 190 pp. Harcourt Brace Jovanovich, Publishers, Orlando, FL 32887.

Offers a firsthand glimpse into the lives of four black women, each of a different generation but all from the same family — all of whom became teenage parents.

Silverstein, Herma. *Teenage and Pregnant: What You Can Do.* 1989. 154 pp. Julian Messner, Silver Burdett Press, 250 James Street, Morristown, NJ 07960. 201/285-7900.

Well-written non-judgmental discussion of the issues facing pregnant teenagers.

Simpson, Carolyn. *Coping with an Unplanned Pregnancy.* 1990. 160 pp. The Rosen Publishing Group, Inc., 29 East 21st Street, New York, NY 10010.

Guide for teenager facing too-early pregnancy. One chapter deals with the possibility of miscarriage or stillbirth—to help the adolescent deal with the grief she is likely to feel if she loses her baby, grief that many people would discount.

Wells, Joel. *Who Do You Think You Are? How to Build Self-Esteem.* 1990. Thomas More, P.O. Box 7000, Allen, TX 75002-1305. 214/390-6325.

This easy-to-read book talks about self-image and building self-esteem. One chapter is titled "The Killing Fields of Adolescence," and deals with the special sensitivity of young people.

Wilson, Olga E. *Coming to Terms.* 124 pp. Afro-In-Books & Things, 5575 N.W. 7th Avenue, Miami, FL 33127. 305/756-6107.

For a candid view of an inner-city unmarried teen mother's life, see this autobiography.

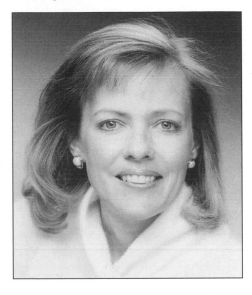

About the Author

Shirley Arthur was a teen mother, and she understands the challenge of teen pregnancy. She shares that understanding with her readers.

Her daughter, Kristina, graduated from the University of Colorado with a bachelor's degree in Journalism, and now works for an advertising agency. Shirley has a B.S. in Business and an M.A. in Communications from the University of Colorado. Her youngest daughter, Kelly, attends Colorado State University.

Shirley works for U S West as a Computer Systems Analyst and Technical Writer. She is also a free-lance writer who enjoys writing for young adults.

She lives in Denver with her husband.

Index

Abortion, 71-79
Abuse, 43
Adoption, 81-91
Adoption agencies, 85-86
Adoption, closed, 83
Adoption costs, 88-89
Adoption, independent, 86-87
Adoption law, 87-88
Adoption, open, 84
AFDC (Aid to Families with
    Dependent Children), 137-138
Agency adoption, 83-85, 87
AIDS, 148-149
Alternatives, 40, 69-115
Bell Jar, The, 69
Birth control, 141-153
Brunelli, Jean, 43
Budget, 136-137
Career planning, 156-159
Child support, 138-139
Childbirth preparation, 66
Childcare, 135-136

Choices, 69-115, 169
Clinic, 39
Closed adoption, 83, 87
Condom, 150
Contraception, 141-153
Counseling, 72, 85-86, 90, 125
Decision making, 105-115
Denial, 54
Depo-Provera, 150
Depression, 74-75
Diaphragm, 150
Do I Have a Daddy? 97
Drugs, 44-46, 61, 66
Education, 139, 155-164, 170
Emotional health, 43, 58, 170
Exercise, 65-66
Family planning, 141-153
Father of baby, 38, 40, 96-99, 112-
    113, 123-126, 133, 138-139,
    164-165
Father's rights, 86
Female condom, 150

Fetal Alcohol Syndrome (FAS), 45, 66
Financial cost, 73
Financial planning, 131-139, 163
Foam, 150
Food pyramid, 64
Friends, 111-112, 121-122
Gibran, Kahlil, 81-82
HUD (Housing and Urban Development) assistance, 138
Independent adoption, 85-86
IUD, 150
Junk food, 65
Life script, 117-118, 167-177
Marriage, 98-99, 134-135
Medical care, 42, 61-62
Meditation, 171
Miscarriage, 41
Movies for the mind, 172-174
New Teenage Body Book, The, 44, 46
Norplant, 150
Nutrition, 58-59, 62-65

Open adoption, 83, 87
Options, 40, 69-115
Parent reactions, 109-111, 134
Parenting, 93-103
Pill, birth control, 150
Plath, Sylvia, 69
Pregnancy test, 38, 39
Presentation ceremony, 91
Prophet, The, 81-82
Rachel, Rachel, 141
Repeat pregnancy, 77-78, 108
Role model, 160-161
Runaway, 42, 44
Self-talk, 174-175
Sexuality, 142-143
Single parent, 94-96
Smoking, 45, 66
Stairway to success, 161
Suicide, 41
Support group, 43
Weight gain, 63-64
WIC (Women, Infant and Children Food Program), 138

OTHER RESOURCES FROM MORNING GLORY PRESS

TEENAGE COUPLES—Caring, Commitment and Change: How to Build a Relationship that Lasts. TEENAGE COUPLES— Coping with Reality: Dealing with Money, In-Laws, Babies and Other Details of Daily Life. Two books to help teenage couples develop healthy, loving and lasting relationships.

TEENAGE COUPLES—Expectations and Reality. For professionals—describes the culture of teenage parents.

TEENS PARENTING—Your Pregnancy and Newborn Journey
How to take care of yourself and your newborn. For pregnant teens. Available in "regular" (RL 6), Easier Reading (RL 3), and Spanish.

TEENS PARENTING—Your Baby's First Year
TEENS PARENTING—The Challenge of Toddlers
TEENS PARENTING—Discipline from Birth to Three
Three how-to-parent books especially for teenage parents.

VIDEOS: "Discipline from Birth to Three" and "Your Baby's First Year" supplement above books.

TEEN DADS: Rights, Responsibilities and Joys. Parenting book for teenage fathers.

DETOUR FOR EMMY. Novel about teenage pregnancy.

TOO SOON FOR JEFF. Novel from teen father's perspective.

TELLING and *BEYOND DREAMS:* More fiction for Young Adults.

SCHOOL-AGE PARENTS: The Challenge of Three-Generation Living. Help for families when teen daughter (or son) has a child.

BREAKING FREE FROM PARTNER ABUSE. Guidance for victims of domestic violence.

DID MY FIRST MOTHER LOVE ME? A Story for an Adopted Child. Birthmother shares her reasons for placing her child.

DO I HAVE A DADDY? A Story About a Single-Parent Child. Picture/story book especially for children with only one parent. Also available in Spanish, *¿Yo tengo papá?*

OPEN ADOPTION: A Caring Option
A fascinating and sensitive account of the new world of adoption.

PARENTS, PREGNANT TEENS AND THE ADOPTION OPTION. For parents of teens considering an adoption plan.

PREGNANT? Adoption Is an Option. Written to help pregnant teens and older women who may be considering an adoption plan.

ADOPTION AWARENESS: A Guide for Teachers, Counselors, Nurses and Caring Others. How to talk about adoption when no one is interested.

MORNING GLORY PRESS

6595 San Haroldo Way, Buena Park, CA 90620
714/828-1998 — FAX 714/828-2049

Please send me the following:　　　　　　　　　　　　Price　　Total

___*Surviving Teen Pregnancy*　Paper, 1-885356-06-4　　11.95 _____
___　　　　　　　　　　　　　　Cloth, 1-885356-05-6　　17.95 _____
　　Teenage Couples: Expectations and Reality
___　　　　　　　　　Paper, ISBN 0-930934-98-9　　14.95 _____
___　　　　　　　　　Cloth, ISBN 0-930934-99-7　　21.95 _____
　　Teenage Couples: Caring, Commitment and Change
___　　　　　　　　　Paper, ISBN 0-930934-93-8　　 9.95 _____
___　　　　　　　　　Cloth, ISBN 0-930934-92-x　　15.95 _____
　　Teenage Couples: Coping with Reality
___　　　　　　　　　Paper, ISBN 0-930934-86-5　　 9.95 _____
___　　　　　　　　　Cloth, ISBN 0930934-87-3　　15.95 _____
___ *Beyond Dreams*　　Paper, ISBN 1-885356-00-5　　 8.95 _____
___*Too Soon for Jeff*　Paper, ISBN 0-930934-91-1　　 8.95 _____
___ *Detour for Emmy*　Paper, ISBN 0-930934-76-8　　 8.95 _____
___*Telling*　　　　　　Paper, ISBN 1-885356-03-x　　 8.95 _____
___*Teen Dads*　　　　　Paper, ISBN 0-930934-78-4　　 9.95 _____
___*Do I Have a Daddy?*　Cloth, ISBN 0-930934-45-8　　12.95 _____
___*Did My First Mother Love Me?* ISBN 0-930934-85-7　12.95 _____
___*Breaking Free from Partner Abuse* 0-930934-74-1　　 7.95 _____
　　School-Age Parents: Three-Generation Living　　　　　　 _____
___　　　　　　　　　Paper, ISBN 0-930934-36-9　　10.95 _____
　　Pregnant? Adoption Is an Option
___　　　　　　　　　Paper, ISBN 1-885356-08-0　　11.95 _____
　　Teens Parenting—Your Pregnancy and Newborn Journey
___　　　　　　　　　Paper, ISBN 0-930934-50-4　　 9.95 _____
　　Spanish—**Adolescentes como padres—La jornada . . .**
___　　　　　　　　　Paper, ISBN 0-930934-69-5　　 9.95 _____
　　Teens Parenting—Your Baby's First Year
___　　　　　　　　　Paper, ISBN 0-930934-52-0　　 9.95 _____
　　Teens Parenting—Challenge of Toddlers
___　　　　　　　　　Paper, ISBN 0-930934-58-x　　 9.95 _____
　　Teens Parenting—Discipline from Birth to Three
___　　　　　　　　　Paper, ISBN 0-930934-54-7　　 9.95 _____
___**VIDEO: "Discipline from Birth to Three"**　　195.00 _____

___**VIDEO: "Your Baby's First Year"**　　　　　195.00 _____

　　　　　　　　　　　　　　　　　　TOTAL　 _____

Please add postage: 10% of total—Min., $3.00　　　　 _____
California residents add 7.75% sales tax
　　　　　　　　　　　　　　　　　　TOTAL　 _____

Ask about quantity discounts, Teacher, Student Guides.
Prepayment requested. School/library purchase orders accepted.
If not satisfied, return in 15 days for refund.

NAME _____

ADDRESS _____

_____